I0885917

Cutting Edge: Your Journey to Becoming a General Surgeon

This book is a practical and comprehensive guide for aspiring surgeons, charting the path from medical school to independent consultant practice. Surgical careers are highly demanding and increasingly competitive, yet many candidates underestimate the challenges and expectations required to succeed. This book aims to bridge that gap by providing clear, structured guidance at every stage of the journey. Whether you are a medical student inspired by a surgical placement, a doctor who has discovered a passion for surgery but is unsure of the next steps, a trainee preparing for consultancy, or a newly appointed consultant looking ahead to the future of the profession, this book offers insight and direction for navigating the realities of a modern surgical career.

The book divides surgical training into three key phases: early, middle, and senior years, providing tailored advice on what to expect, how to maximise training opportunities, and how to build a competitive portfolio at each stage. Readers will gain invaluable insights on strengthening applications, optimising placements, developing leadership and academic experience, and approaching increasingly competitive selection processes with confidence and foresight.

Beyond technical and clinical training, *Cutting Edge: Your Journey to Becoming a General Surgeon* also explores the broader realities of contemporary surgical practice. Dedicated chapters address topics such as diversity and inclusion, emotional resilience, surgery in the age of social media, and the future direction of the profession, reflecting the challenges and opportunities faced by today's surgeons. Designed for medical students, surgical trainees, and doctors approaching independent consultant practice, this book also serves as a valuable resource for international medical graduates seeking to understand training pathways, as well as for surgical educators, mentors, and programme directors supporting the next generation of surgeons.

Cutting Edge: Your Journey to Becoming a General Surgeon

Sala Abdalla BSc MBBS FRCS (Gen Surg) FEBS AWS
London North West University Healthcare NHS Trust, London, UK

Karen Chien Lin Soh MBBChir MA (Cantab) MRCS
Imperial College Healthcare NHS Trust, London, UK

CRC Press
Taylor & Francis Group
Boca Raton London New York

CRC Press is an imprint of the
Taylor & Francis Group, an **informa** business

Designed cover image: Shutterstock

First edition published 2027
by CRC Press
2385 NW Executive Center Drive, Suite 320, Boca Raton FL 33431

and by CRC Press
4 Park Square, Milton Park, Abingdon, Oxon, OX14 4RN

CRC Press is an imprint of Taylor & Francis Group, LLC

ISBN: 978-1-032-88419-6 (hbk)
ISBN: 978-1-032-88293-2 (pbk)
ISBN: 978-1-003-53766-3 (ebk)

DOI: 10.1201/9781003537663

Typeset in Minion
by SPi Technologies India Pvt Ltd (Straive)

Contents

About the authors

Miss Sala Abdalla BSc MBBS FRCS (Gen Surg) is a Consultant General and Upper Gastrointestinal Surgeon based in London. She is a graduate of Imperial College, London, and has completed her specialist surgical training at several internationally renowned teaching hospitals across the capital. She is widely recognised for her longstanding commitment to surgical education and mentorship of trainees at all stages of their careers, both within the United Kingdom and internationally. She plays an active role in postgraduate education through her involvement with the London School of Surgery, the Royal College of Surgeons of England, and a range of national and international educational initiatives.

Beyond her clinical and educational work, Miss Abdalla is deeply committed to improving equitable access to safe surgical care worldwide. She serves as Managing Director of Operation International UK, a charitable surgical organisation that has worked in close partnership with the Royal College of Surgeons of England to deliver sustainable, life-changing surgical care in underserved and resource-limited settings.

Drawing on her clinical experience, educational leadership, and global health work, Miss Abdalla brings a unique and informed perspective to this manual. Her aim is to educate, empower, and inspire the next generation of surgeons.

Miss Karen Chien Lin Soh MBBChir MA (Cantab) MRCS is a Core Surgical Trainee in the London deanery with a clinical focus in general and vascular surgery. She graduated with distinction from the University of Cambridge, where she also completed an intercalated degree in Manufacturing Engineering. Her diverse experience spans clinical settings across the United Kingdom, the United States, and Asia, complemented by a strong background in non-clinical fields, including management consulting, finance, and translational research. Through her contributions to this manual, Miss Soh aims to offer a valuable early career perspective for aspiring general surgeons, drawing on both her clinical and interdisciplinary experience.

Foreword: Professor Dame Averil Mansfield FRCS

The most important and difficult decision you will make in your life is to become a surgeon. If you are still undecided, then this book will assist you in that decision, supplementing your personal visits and contacts with surgeons and surgical units.

For those of you who have already made the decision to become a surgeon, this book is for you.

It will give you a detailed guide to all the steps you need to take in order to make progress in that career choice.

Starting with steps you can take right from the beginning of your life as a student and then resident doctor, it will inform you of all that is available, all that is optional, and all that is required. It will help you to build a Curriculum Vitae (CV) that is competitive.

Knowledge of such building blocks is difficult to acquire by an individual who is starting out in surgery. With this guide, you will find the confidence to plan and make effective progress. Throughout your training, there are decisions and choices to be made, and you can learn of these here and be assisted in how to approach those next steps.

This is not simply an outline of what is needed to make progress but a detailed source book of where to find the information you will need. The authors have provided you with a straightforward and informative route map which will be invaluable.

It goes well beyond the building blocks of a career but also addresses some of the problems and difficulties and human frailties that you may encounter on the way and will help to find a way through these.

To those of you setting out on this road to a surgical career, I wish you success and the happiness that I experienced. We are privileged in being entrusted with the surgical care of our fellow human beings. This book will enable you to gain that trust and also to care for yourself.

Professor Dame Averil Mansfield FRCS
Emeritus professor of vascular surgery

Foreword: Miss Hannah Maple FRCS PhD

As the first medic in my family, I was extremely naïve when I decided I wanted to pursue a career in medicine, let alone become a surgeon. It is only in my latter years of training, and now as I reflect as a consultant, that I realise how disadvantaged I was by not having the right friends or relatives in the right places. I was unaware of the training pathway, the challenges I would face and the obstacles that would be put in my way.

Without access to people on the inside, for my generation there was very little guidance on how to plan a surgical career, how to manage issues such as racial and sexual discrimination, and how to evolve into the surgeon I wanted to become. I was very fortunate to hold hands with, and be inspired by, some amazing friends and mentors, but like many women of my generation, I had to do it the hard way.

This book, which is lovingly and expertly put together, is the book I wish I'd had when I decided to become a general surgeon. Crucially, it levels the playing field for the underdog, i.e., those of you who, like me, may at one point have thought that surgery is not for someone like them. It provides the reader with a roadmap of what is to come with a detailed description of every career stage, alongside guidance on all the things you've not even thought about yet. Whilst the focus is on a career in general surgery, I would urge surgeons at any stage of their careers to give it a read, regardless of speciality, to ensure that surgery really can be a career for anyone who is dedicated enough to pursue it.

Miss Hannah Maple FRCS PhD
Consultant Transplant and Dialysis Access Surgeon

Preface

Being a surgeon is immeasurably rewarding. There is nothing more satisfying than seeing your patients' lives transformed for the better after a surgical intervention. Every surgery is an adventure, filled with the consoling, practiced sense of the known and the anticipation and exhilaration of the unknown. Surgeons would tell you that they experience tremendous satisfaction in solving problems by combining their knowledge with technical prowess.

Surgery is widely regarded as one of the most challenging and respected medical specialties, demanding unwavering commitment, discipline, and a dedication to lifelong learning. Surgical excellence is not innate but achieved through perseverance, purposeful training, and a strong work ethic. General surgery, with its wide-ranging clinical scope and technical complexity, offers a uniquely stimulating and fulfilling career. It unites the intellectual rigour of diagnostic reasoning with the tangible impact of operative care, allowing surgeons to make a direct and meaningful difference to patients' lives. Beyond clinical practice, the field offers abundant opportunities for innovation, research, education, and global health engagement, empowering surgeons to shape the future of healthcare and lead change within the profession.

Early preparation towards a career in general surgery is essential and can begin as early as medical school. Across the United Kingdom (UK), undergraduate surgical societies play a pivotal role in supporting aspiring surgeons by organising conferences, workshops, and skills sessions that offer valuable insights into the realities of a surgical career.

In the early postgraduate years, targeted clinical placements in surgical specialties, attendance at relevant courses and conferences, and access to experienced mentors can further enhance understanding and enthusiasm for the profession. These opportunities offer a meaningful glimpse into the surgical field and help lay the foundation for a successful and informed entry into core surgical training.

The UK surgical training pathway is widely regarded as one of the most comprehensive and respected in the world. While it is a lengthy and demanding journey, it remains one of the most sought-after routes globally for those aspiring to a career in surgery. Entry into both core and higher surgical training is highly competitive, requiring success in national selection processes that include a detailed formal application and a structured interview. These assessments evaluate a candidate's surgical portfolio, clinical acumen, and management skills. In an increasingly competitive landscape, the key to success in entering specialist surgical training lies in early and meticulous preparation.

Contemporary general surgical practice and training have in recent decades undergone substantial change, shaping both the opportunities available to trainees and the challenges they face. Surgical training continues to demand resilience, adaptability, and sustained motivation, as individuals navigate intense competition, the financial burden of examinations and mandatory courses, and an increasingly complex clinical workload. Evolving working patterns, including shorter and more fragmented apprenticeship hours, have prompted reflection on how surgical skills are acquired and how continuity of patient care is maintained. Long and often unpredictable working hours, demanding on-call commitments, and expectations to contribute to research, teaching, and administrative activities can accumulate over time, leading to physical fatigue and emotional strain. While the growing diversity of the surgical workforce is a welcome and necessary development, it has also brought renewed attention to the persistent challenges of unconscious bias, discrimination, and systemic inequality. The COVID-19 global pandemic further highlighted vulnerabilities within the training environment, disrupting hands-on learning and intensifying stress and burnout among trainees. In parallel, the influence of social media and rapidly evolving technologies reflects an ever-changing surgical landscape, offering new opportunities for learning and collaboration while also introducing additional pressures and complexities.

In light of these realities, preparing for a career in surgery involves more than academic and clinical excellence; it requires physical stamina, emotional intelligence, and strategies to manage the inevitable obstacles that arise along the way.

This manual is designed to guide the aspiring surgeon through the entire continuum of training, from medical school through to the transition into consultant practice. It offers practical advice on building a strong surgical portfolio, maximising opportunities during foundation and core training, and making the most of out-of-programme experiences. Dedicated sections provide insights into progressing through training and assessments, protecting time for professional development, and honing non-technical skills such as leadership, communication, and decision-making. The UK surgical training curriculum is rigorous and clearly defined, with high standards that must be met to achieve the Certificate of Completion of Training (CCT). Successful completion of this pathway marks the beginning of a new phase: independent practice as a consultant surgeon. An entire chapter in this book is dedicated to supporting new consultants as they prepare for this transition, offering guidance on the responsibilities, expectations, and opportunities that come with senior clinical roles. Importantly, additional chapters importantly focus on the practical and emotional challenges frequently encountered during training, offering thoughtful discussion on how to navigate setbacks, respond to unexpected changes, and seek support when needed.

This book is intended not only as a practical resource but also as a source of inspiration. It aims to energise and empower future surgeons, offering a structured roadmap through the surgical training journey, from the first steps in medical school to the threshold of independent consultant practice.

Acknowledgements

I want to express my heartfelt gratitude to my family and to the many colleagues, past and present, who have inspired me. The insights I've gained over the years have shaped my journey, and it's a privilege to now contribute to the development of those just beginning theirs.

Sala Abdalla BSc MBBS FRCS (Gen Surg) FEBS AWS

Thank you to my family, friends, and colleagues for their unconditional support.

Karen Chien Lin Soh MBBChir MA (Cantab) MRCS

1

Introduction: The speciality of general surgery

WHAT IS GENERAL SURGERY IN THE UK TODAY?

General surgery is a broad surgical specialty focussed on the operative and non-operative management of abdominal, visceral, and related conditions. In the United Kingdom (UK), it remains one of the largest and most diverse surgical disciplines, forming the backbone of acute surgical care within the National Health Service (NHS). While the title "general" suggests breadth, modern general surgery is best understood as a generalist framework with increasing subspecialisation. General surgery has witnessed significant transformation as a speciality since its inception, and continues to be shaped by rapid advancements in healthcare and technology.

Most UK general surgeons develop a subspecialty interest during higher surgical or specialist training. Major subspecialties include colorectal surgery, upper gastrointestinal surgery (UGI), hepatopancreaticobiliary (HPB) surgery, breast surgery, endocrine surgery, and transplant surgery. Subspecialisation reflects the increasing complexity in surgical care, advances in technology, and the need for high procedural volumes to maintain expertise. Even highly subspecialised consultants are expected to contribute to the emergency general surgery rota, particularly in District General Hospitals (DGHs). General surgeons are often the front-line of call for acute surgical problems, acting as first responders for conditions requiring immediate life-saving intervention and stabilisation. This dual identity: specialist by day, generalist on call, is a defining feature of the UK general surgeon (Figure 1.1).

DOI: 10.1201/9781003537663-1

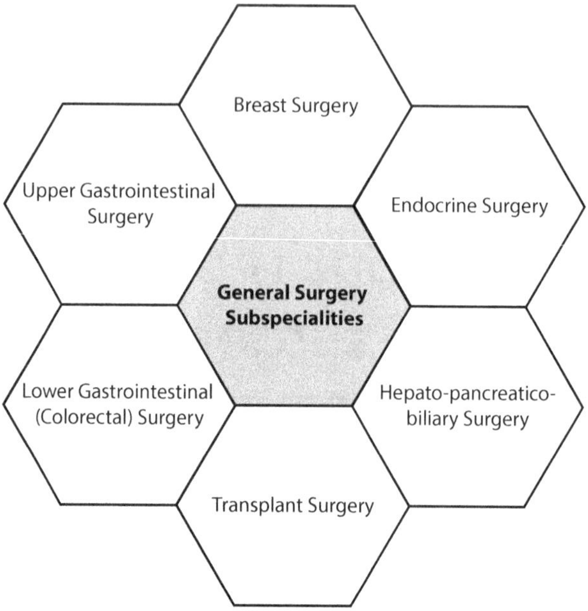

Figure 1.1 Diagram depicting subspecialities within general surgery.

SCOPE OF PRACTICE: EMERGENCY AND ELECTIVE SURGERY

UK general surgeons typically divide their workload between emergency and elective practice. Emergency general surgery (EGS) includes the assessment and management of acutely unwell patients presenting with acute gastrointestinal conditions such as appendicitis, bowel obstruction/perforation, intra-abdominal sepsis, gastrointestinal bleeding, and abdominal trauma. This work is unpredictable, time-pressured, and often undertaken out of hours, thereby requiring rapid decision-making under conditions of uncertainty. Beyond surgical management of emergency conditions, EGS also involves daily inpatient care including decisions regarding admissions and discharges, collaboration with the multidisciplinary team, and the provision of surgical advice to community teams, emergency departments, and other inpatient care teams.

Elective general surgery, by contrast, involves planned procedures such as hernia repair, cholecystectomy, colorectal resections, and cancer surgery. Elective practice allows for more detailed preoperative planning, multidisciplinary discussion, and longitudinal patient care. Elective care also includes the provision of outpatient clinic services and the assessment of patients referred from community services with general surgical conditions. In comparison to EGS, elective general surgery requires planning over a longer period of time, often working in collaboration with other surgical or non-surgical specialities.

Most consultants practise a combination of both emergency and elective general surgery, although the balance varies depending on subspecialty, hospital setting, and job plan.

DISTRICT GENERAL HOSPITALS VERSUS TERTIARY CENTRES

The nature of general surgical practice can vary between DGHs and tertiary referral centres, reflecting differences in the case mix, service configuration, and availability of subspecialist support. In DGH settings, general surgeons typically provide emergency and elective services, managing a broad spectrum of common and acute surgical conditions. This often includes the assessment and treatment of unselected emergency admissions, routine elective procedures, and, in many cases, emergency oncological resections.

Consultants working in DGHs are frequently required to maintain a wide skill set and a high degree of clinical autonomy, as subspecialist cover may be limited or unavailable on-site. When patients present with complex pathology or require highly specialised interventions beyond the scope of local services, DGH consultants routinely collaborate with colleagues in tertiary referral centres. This collaboration may involve seeking subspecialist advice, shared decision-making regarding optimal management, or arranging the transfer of patients to tertiary centres for intervention or ongoing care. Such integrated working relationships are essential to ensuring the delivery of high-quality care and equitable access to specialist services.

In contrast, tertiary referral centres are structured to manage higher volumes of complex and specialist surgical cases, often serving as regional or national hubs for advanced care. These centres typically offer a greater concentration of subspecialist expertise, access to specialised multidisciplinary teams, and advanced diagnostic and interventional resources. As a result, surgical practice in tertiary settings is more focussed on complex elective work, high-risk emergency surgery, and the management of patients with rare or advanced pathology.

The interaction between DGHs and tertiary referral centres is therefore a fundamental component of modern surgical service delivery. For surgeons, this collaborative model supports safe decision-making, appropriate escalation of care, and shared responsibility for complex cases.

For trainees, exposure to both DGH and tertiary centre environments is invaluable, offering complementary learning experiences. Training in DGHs promotes the development of broad-based surgical competence, independent decision-making, and confidence in managing unselected emergency workloads, while time spent in tertiary centres provides experience in subspecialist practice and exposure to advanced surgical techniques and research opportunities. Together, these settings contribute to the development of well-rounded general surgeons equipped to practise safely and effectively across diverse healthcare environments.

FROM BARBER-SURGEONS TO MODERN SPECIALISTS

Historically, general surgeons were truly "general," managing conditions that now fall under orthopaedics, neurosurgery, vascular surgery, and paediatrics. As early as Ancient Egypt, surgeons 'managed' surgical conditions by surgical conditions through setting bone fractures, removing tumours, and managing wounds. These surgical practices continued through Ancient Greece and Rome, where foundational principles of surgical education and clinical observation were established by figures such as Hippocrates.

Moving forward into the medieval and Tudor periods, surgeons were barbers by trade, with no formal medical training, and performed basic surgical procedures using the same sharp tools they used for haircuts and shaving. Barbers and surgeons became inextricably linked in 1540 when the Barber-Surgeons Company began to regulate these basic surgical procedures. In 1745, as surgical practice evolved further, this company was split by Parliament, eventually culminating in the development of the modern Royal College of Surgeons of England. This heritage persists symbolically in the continued use of the titles Mr and Ms/Miss/Mrs, a legacy of the barber-surgeon era before formal medical training was introduced for surgeons.

With the advent of anaesthesia, asepsis and modern surgical techniques, the practice of surgery has transformed significantly far beyond its initial origins.

BECOMING A GENERAL SURGEON IN THE UK

The UK traditional training pathway to consultancy

Becoming a consultant general surgeon in the UK can follow several pathways, each offering different timelines, structures, and experiences.

These routes are overseen by national regulatory and training bodies, such as the General Medical Council (GMC), the NHS, Health Education England/Scotland/Wales, and the Intercollegiate Surgical Curriculum Programme (ISCP), with significant input from the Royal Colleges of Surgeons (RCS) and other professional organisations.

The most common pathway begins after graduation from medical school with the two-year Foundation Programme, followed by two years of Core Surgical Training. This is then succeeded by approximately six years of Specialty Training in general surgery. Once a Certificate of Completion of Training (CCT) is achieved, a locum or substantive consultant post can be sought where available. Progression between each stage is competitive, and trainees may choose to take time out of the training programme at various stages to pursue research degrees, international fellowships, leadership roles, or other professional interests (Figure 1.2).

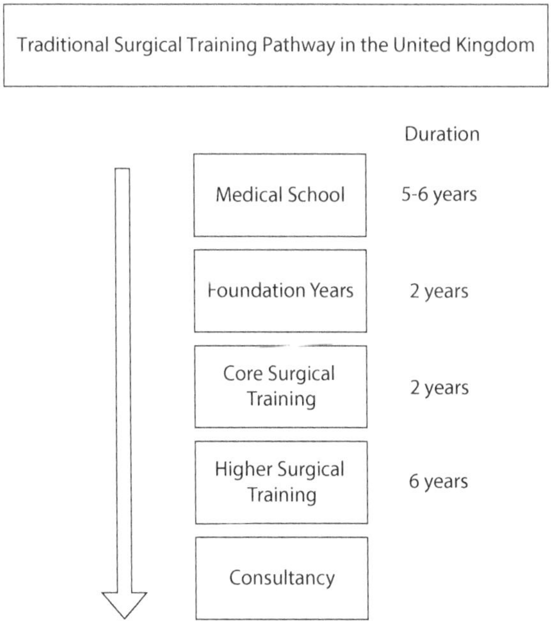

Figure 1.2 Flowchart for traditional training pathway.

Alternative pathways for international medical graduates to consultancy or specialty roles

As the surgical workforce becomes increasingly globalised, the UK has developed a range of structured pathways to support international medical graduates (IMGs) seeking to enter and progress within the profession. These routes recognise the diverse training backgrounds and clinical experience of surgeons from around the world, while ensuring that standards of practice remain aligned with those required for independent consultant practice in the UK.

One such pathway is the Certificate of Eligibility for Specialist Registration (CESR), which provides an alternative route to consultant appointment for surgeons who have not completed a UK-approved CCT programme. The CESR pathway has grown steadily in popularity in recent years, reflecting both workforce demands and an increasing number of experienced international surgeons seeking recognition of their competencies within the UK system. A subtype of the CESR pathway, the CESR-Combined Programme (CESR-CP) applies to doctors who complete part of their specialty training within a UK-approved training programme but do not follow the full CCT route. While both pathways lead to entry onto the GMC Specialist Register, CESR requires retrospective demonstration of equivalence to UK training through a comprehensive evidence portfolio, whereas CESR-CP involves prospectively assessed training with defined competencies achieved during an approved programme.

Through the CESR process, applicants are required to demonstrate that their training, experience, and professional development are equivalent in scope and standard to those of a UK-trained consultant. This involves the submission of comprehensive evidence mapped against the relevant specialty curriculum, encompassing clinical competence, operative experience, leadership, education, research, governance, and professional behaviours. While the process is rigorous and documentation-intensive, it provides a transparent and robust mechanism for recognising equivalence and supporting workforce integration.

The expansion of routes such as CESR highlights the UK's commitment to maintaining high clinical standards while embracing the benefits of a diverse and internationally trained surgical workforce (Figure 1.3).

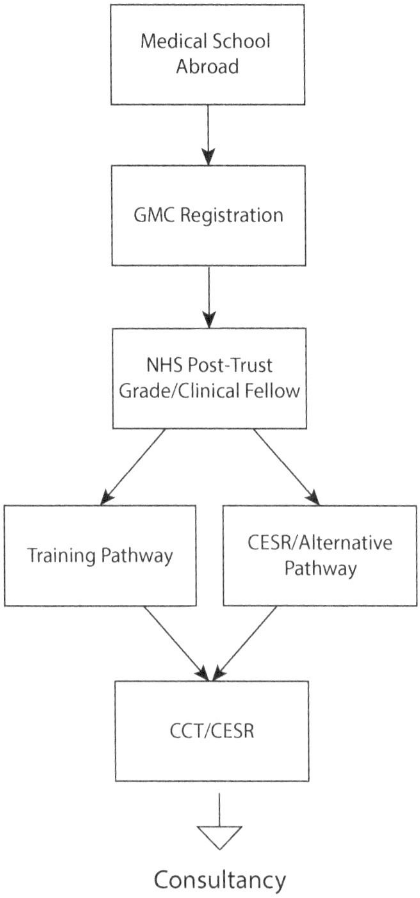

Figure 1.3 Flowchart for alternative pathway for IMG to consultancy.

Not all IMGs aspire to consultant-level practice. For a variety of personal and professional reasons, some IMGs choose to pursue careers as specialty doctors rather than seeking consultant appointments, which are associated with broader clinical scope and significant non-clinical responsibilities. Speciality roles offer an alternative career pathway that allows doctors to focus on defined areas of clinical practice and contribute meaningfully to service delivery while achieving a balance that aligns with individual career goals and circumstances (Figure 1.4).

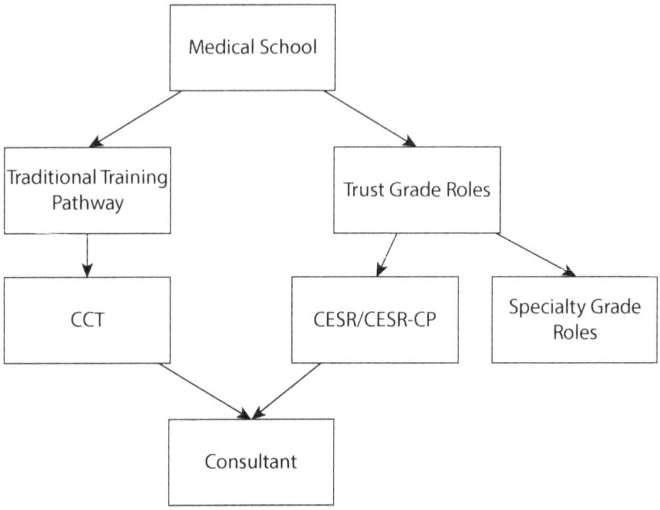

Figure 1.4 Flowchart for traditional and CESR/CESR-CP pathways to consultancy. CCT – Certificate of Completion of Training; CESR-CP – Certificate of Eligibility for Specialist Registration Combined Programme; CESR – Certificate of Eligibility for Specialist Registration.

EVOLUTION OF GENERAL SURGERY IN THE UK AND BEYOND

General surgery, like the rest of modern medicine, has undergone remarkable transformation over the past century. Continuous scientific innovation and international collaboration have accelerated the development of new tools and techniques designed to improve patient outcomes. Contemporary general surgeons must master a range of advanced skills, particularly in minimally invasive surgery. Laparoscopic techniques, once novel, are now standard practice, enabling faster recovery and reduced post-operative pain. Robotic surgery is also expanding rapidly, especially within colorectal, upper gastrointestinal, abdominal wall and surgical specialties, offering enhanced precision and ergonomics for complex operations.

Surgical training itself is evolving in parallel. Simulation-based education, virtual reality, and augmented reality are increasingly integrated into training programmes, providing safe and sophisticated environments for practising operative skills. Emerging artificial intelligence tools are beginning to support clinical decision-making, streamline workflows, and enhance both patient and surgeon education. Surgery as a field is ever changing, and aspiring surgeons must keep up to date with the latest developments to transform with the field.

CHALLENGES FACING THE MODERN GENERAL SURGEON

The scope of general surgery is evolving rapidly, and today's surgeons must navigate an array of complex challenges shaped by demographic shifts, technological progress, and global pressures. These forces are transforming not only the clinical demands placed on surgeons, but also the broader cultural context in which surgical care is delivered.

One of the most significant challenges arises from an ageing population with increasingly complex comorbidities. Advances in medical care have extended lifespans, but they have also introduced a growing cohort of patients who present with multiple chronic conditions. This leads to a higher volume of surgical referrals and a marked increase in the complexity of perioperative decision-making. Managing frailty, polypharmacy, cardiopulmonary disease, and other age-related issues has become an integral part of surgical practice.

Alongside this demographic shift, rising rates of obesity across both adult and paediatric populations pose additional technical and clinical difficulties. Obesity is associated with higher perioperative risk and more technically demanding operations, often requiring advanced laparoscopic or robotic approaches. It also contributes to the growing burden of metabolic, hepatobiliary, and gastrointestinal pathologies, further increasing demand on surgical services. At the system level, the challenge of finite resources remains a persistent and global concern. Workforce shortages, including an insufficient number of trained surgeons, are contributing to expanding waiting lists and delayed access to care. Infrastructure limitations, uneven distribution of specialist services, and financial pressures compound the strain on healthcare systems worldwide.

The COVID-19 global pandemic of 2020 was a seismic event that underscored the vulnerability of surgical services to external shocks. Elective surgery backlogs, disrupted training, and heightened pressure on emergency services revealed the need for adaptable, resilient systems capable of withstanding future crises, whether infectious, economic, or geopolitical.

Environmental sustainability has also become a pressing issue. Climate change has intensified scrutiny of the carbon footprint and resource use associated with surgical practice. This has led to growing interest in "green surgery": adopting sustainable materials, optimising energy use, reducing waste, and rethinking the design of operating theatres to align with global environmental goals.

Modern general surgeons must therefore balance high-quality clinical care with the realities of rising demand, limited resources, public health challenges, and environmental responsibility. The profession is being reshaped not only by what surgeons can do but also by what society needs them to do, today and in the decades ahead.

NHS REALITIES VERSUS PUBLIC PERCEPTION

Public perception often portrays surgeons as theatre-based technicians performing dramatic life-saving operations. This is often through portrayals in popular media, such as television shows and books. In reality, the NHS general surgeon's role is far broader and increasingly constrained by systemic pressures. Significant time is spent on ward rounds, outpatient clinics, multidisciplinary meetings, administrative tasks, and service delivery planning. Rising waiting lists, bed pressures, rota gaps, and workforce shortages have become daily realities.

While surgery remains a hands-on specialty, modern consultants must also function as leaders, managers and educators within a stretched healthcare system. Understanding this reality early is essential for anyone considering the specialty.

IS GENERAL SURGERY THE RIGHT CAREER FOR YOU?

Choosing a career in general surgery requires a level of honest self-reflection that extends beyond academic ability or technical aptitude. The specialty suits individuals who are comfortable making decisions in high-pressure environments and accepting responsibility for outcomes that are often rapid but not always favourable. Surgeons frequently work with incomplete information, manage uncertainty, and must act decisively while remaining open to input from colleagues. Traits such as resilience, practicality, and adaptability are essential, and while a degree of perfectionism can drive high standards, it must be tempered by humility, self-awareness, and an ability to function effectively within a multidisciplinary team.

The demands of surgery are not solely intellectual. The physical nature of the work includes long operating lists, extended periods of standing, and the cumulative fatigue associated with on-call duties. Emotional resilience is equally important. Surgeons must navigate complications, unexpected outcomes, and challenging conversations with patients and families, sometimes in the context of severe illness or death. Cognitively, the role requires sustained concentration, rapid assimilation of complex information, and a commitment to lifelong learning as techniques, evidence, and technologies continue to evolve.

Lifestyle considerations also warrant careful thought. Although working conditions have profoundly improved, general surgery remains a specialty defined by shift work, overnight on-call commitments, weekend duties, and the inherent unpredictability of emergency care. Achieving a satisfactory work-life balance is possible, but it is not effortless and is influenced by factors such as hospital setting, subspecialty focus, and career stage.

It is equally important to recognise when surgery may not be the right fit. Individuals who strongly value predictable working hours, lower-intensity decision-making, or minimal exposure to acute clinical pressure may find the demands of surgery difficult to reconcile with their personal priorities. Discomfort with procedural work or high-stakes responsibility are also legitimate reasons to pursue alternative paths. Medicine offers a wide range of rewarding careers, and choosing not to enter surgery reflects thoughtful self-assessment rather than failure.

WHY CHOOSE A CAREER IN GENERAL SURGERY?

General surgery is a deeply rewarding specialty, one that attracts individuals who thrive in fast-paced environments and are motivated by meaningful, hands-on patient care. No two days are alike. A surgeon may move from managing critically ill patients on the ward, to performing emergency operations, to conducting planned elective procedures, each requiring precision, adaptability, and sound clinical judgement.

The challenges are significant, but so too are the rewards. Few careers offer the privilege of intervening so directly in moments of acute illness, relieving pain, preventing life-threatening complications, and saving lives outright. The satisfaction of restoring health through skilled operative intervention forms the foundation of what many surgeons describe as the most fulfilling aspect of their work.

General surgery also offers exceptional opportunities for academic growth and innovation. As surgical techniques, technologies, and care pathways evolve, surgeons can engage in research that shapes the future of the field, from minimally invasive approaches and robotics to biomaterials and artificial intelligence. For those with a passion for discovery, teaching, or leadership, the specialty provides ample scope to develop a rich and varied professional life.

In addition to the intellectual and clinical rewards, the career can bring financial stability, and long-term career satisfaction. Yet, the decision to pursue general surgery must be a thoughtful and personal one.

It requires honest reflection on one's interests, values, and willingness to commit to a career that is both highly demanding and profoundly impactful.

For those who seek challenge, purpose, and the opportunity to make a tangible difference, general surgery can offer an extraordinarily meaningful path.

BIBLIOGRAPHY

BMJ. The Complete Guide to Becoming a General Surgeon [Internet]. *BMJ Careers*. 2023. Available from: https://www.bmj.com/careers/article/the-complete-guide-to-becoming-a-general-surgeon-

Gawande A. Two hundred years of surgery. *The New England Journal of Medicine*. 2012 May 3;366(18):1716–1723. doi:10.1056/NEJMra1202392. Erratum in: N Engl J Med. 2012 Aug 9;367(6):582. PMID: 22551130.

General Medical Council. Outcomes for graduates [Internet]. www.gmc-uk.org. 2020. Available from: https://www.gmc-uk.org/education/standards-guidance-and-curricula/standards-and-outcomes/outcomes-for-graduates/outcomes-for-graduates

General Medical Council. General surgery curriculum [Internet]. Gmc-uk.org. 2024 [cited 2024 Nov 12]. Available from: https://www.gmc-uk.org/education/standards-guidance-and-curricula/curricula/general-surgery-curriculum

Health Education England. General Surgery | London [Internet]. Hee.nhs.uk. 2018 [cited 2024 Nov 12]. Available from: https://london.hee.nhs.uk/specialty-schools/surgery/general-surgery

McKellar S. A history of surgery: From superstition to science. *CMAJ*. 2010 May 18;182(8):809. doi:10.1503/cmaj.100436. PMCID: PMC2871217.

NHS. General surgery [Internet]. *Health Careers*. 2015. Available from: https://www.healthcareers.nhs.uk/explore-roles/doctors/roles-doctors/surgery/general-surgery

NHS England. Applying | Workforce, training and education | NHS England [Internet]. NHS England | Workforce, training and education | Medical Hub. 2024 [cited 2024 Nov 12]. Available from: https://medical.hee.nhs.uk/medical-training-recruitment/medical-specialty-training/surgery/higher-surgery/general-surgery/overview-of-general-surgery/how-to-apply

Payne T, Toms JD, Zaidi A, Thrumurthy SG. The history of surgery and surgical training in the UK. *Pakistan Journal of Medical Sciences*. 2021 Sep–Oct;37(5):1532–1535. doi:10.12669/pjms.37.5.4628. PMID: 34475943; PMCID: PMC8377927.

RCS England. How to get ahead in surgery [Internet]. Royal College of Surgeons. Available from: https://www.rcseng.ac.uk/careers-in-surgery/trainees/foundation-and-core-trainees/how-to-get-ahead-in-surgery/

RCS England. Surgical specialties — Royal College of Surgeons [Internet]. Royal College of Surgeons. 2016. Available from: https://www.rcseng.ac.uk/careers-in-surgery/trainees/foundation-and-core-trainees/surgical-specialties/

RCS England. Surgical training in the UK — Royal College of Surgeons [Internet]. Royal College of Surgeons. 2024b. Available from: https://www.rcseng.ac.uk/careers-in-surgery/international-trainees-and-surgeons/uk-surgical-training/

RCS England. What is surgery like as a career? – Royal College of Surgeons [Internet]. Royal College of Surgeons. 2024a [cited 2024 Nov 12]. Available from: https://www.rcseng.ac.uk/careers-in-surgery/careers-support/what-is-surgery-like-as-a-career/?gad_source=1&gclid=Cj0KCQiAoae5BhCNARIsADVLzZcTSdcwutX-POCuuxJqzNBx_iLVuXHzexluM2PZsPBSovRpol3kTEkaAtiPEALw_wcB

2

The early years: Medical school

INTRODUCTION

The aspiration to pursue a career in general surgery often begins early, sometimes as early as medical school. This formative period offers a unique opportunity to explore the specialty, with an ever-expanding range of resources and experiences now available to introduce students to surgery at an undergraduate level. Meaningful exposure, whether through clinical rotations, surgical societies, or encounters with inspiring surgeons who serve as role models, can be pivotal in shaping a student's professional ambitions and fostering a lasting interest in general surgery.

Opportunities such as intercalated bachelor's degrees with a surgical focus and elective placements in general surgery allow students to engage more deeply with the specialty, offering insight into its intellectual challenge, technical skill, and patient impact. Equally important is the process of self-reflection: considering one's personal attributes, motivations, and long-term aspirations is essential when contemplating a career that is both demanding and deeply rewarding.

This chapter aims to guide readers in making the most of their medical school years as they begin to prepare for a future in general surgery. As one of the largest and most competitive surgical specialties in the UK, general surgery requires early engagement, thoughtful planning, and sustained commitment. By recognising and embracing opportunities from the outset, aspiring surgeons can lay a strong foundation for a fulfilling career.

DOI: 10.1201/9781003537663-2

DESIRABLE PERSONAL QUALITIES

There is no single profile or "ideal" individual suited to a career in general surgery. The UK general surgical workforce is increasingly diverse, enriched by a broad range of backgrounds, perspectives, and experiences. What unites general surgeons is not a uniform personality but a shared set of values and qualities that support excellence in a challenging and dynamic specialty.

At its core, general surgery appeals to those who are curious and driven by problem-solving. General surgeons are frequently required to think critically and adapt swiftly, particularly when faced with unexpected situations in the operating theatre. The specialty demands the ability to remain calm and composed in high-pressure environments while maintaining clear, compassionate communication with patients, their families, and the multidisciplinary team. As with all areas of medicine, empathy and strong interpersonal skills are fundamental to delivering high-quality patient care.

General surgery also attracts individuals who are hardworking and resilient, with the physical and mental stamina required to meet the long hours and intense demands of surgical practice. As a hands-on specialty, it requires an interest in developing technical skills and manual dexterity, skills that are cultivated through sustained practice and commitment. Medical students considering surgery should be willing to immerse themselves in learning, embracing both challenge and continuous improvement.

Equally important is a commitment to lifelong learning and professional development, as the field of surgery continues to evolve. Above all, passion for the specialty and the determination to persevere through setbacks are qualities that sustain surgeons throughout their careers. While these attributes are not prerequisites, they provide a strong foundation for those aspiring to build a fulfilling and enduring career in general surgery.

SURGICAL PLACEMENTS: MAKING THE MOST OF YOUR EXPERIENCE

Surgical placements represent a pivotal stage in medical training, offering students their first exposure to the realities of surgical practice. In many traditional medical schools, these placements begin during the clinical years, often from the third year onwards, while newer curricula may introduce surgical experiences earlier in the first and second years to enhance clinical immersion. Where choice is available, students with an interest in surgery are encouraged to tailor their placements towards surgical specialties, including general surgery and its subspecialties. Exposure to a broad range of general surgical disciplines is invaluable, helping students develop a realistic understanding of the specialty and refine their future career aspirations. Many surgeons cite these early encounters as formative, shaping both their professional identity and long-term ambitions.

Surgical placements are typically undertaken in blocks lasting several weeks and provide insight into the full spectrum of surgical care. Students may participate in outpatient clinics, ward rounds, multidisciplinary meetings, and operating theatre sessions, gaining an appreciation of how surgical teams function across different clinical environments. Beyond technical learning, these placements foster professionalism and interprofessional collaboration, as students work closely with surgeons, nurses, anaesthetists, and allied healthcare professionals to deliver patient-centred care.

The operating theatre, though initially intimidating, offers rich opportunities for learning and skill development. Preparation is key to maximising this experience. Reviewing operating lists in advance, familiarising oneself with patients' clinical histories, and understanding the indications for surgery enable students to engage more meaningfully with procedures. Observing pre-operative assessment and how patients are pre-optimised for surgery, particularly patients with complex medical conditions, provides valuable insight into surgical decision-making and holistic patient care.

Complementing clinical exposure with independent study is essential, as it enhances the learning. Revising relevant anatomy, surgical principles, and the key steps of procedures allows students to contextualise what they observe and consolidate knowledge. Teaching sessions led by surgeons are an important component of placements and are most effective when supported by pre-reading and self-directed learning. A wide range of educational resources, including textbooks and reputable online platforms, can help deepen understanding beyond the undergraduate curriculum.

Active participation of students in the operating theatre is strongly encouraged. Learning to scrub, practising knot-tying, and developing familiarity with theatre etiquette demonstrate initiative and enthusiasm. Attendance at recognised surgical skills courses can help students build confidence and acquire foundational technical skills, enabling them to take greater advantage of opportunities during placements. Surgical learning is both observational and experiential, and motivated students may be invited to assist with tasks such as wound closure or basic procedures under supervision.

Building professional relationships within the surgical team enhances both learning and enjoyment. Engaging with the lead surgeon, resident doctors and theatre staff fosters trust and opens doors to teaching opportunities. Students should feel encouraged to ask questions and remain curious, recognising that mistakes are an expected and valuable part of the learning process. Reflecting on feedback and following up on unfamiliar topics helps reinforce knowledge and supports continuous improvement.

Participating in clinical sessions outside the operating theatre is equally important. Following patients through clinics, wards, and emergency admissions provides a comprehensive view of the surgical journey, from initial assessment to post-operative care. Active involvement in ward rounds and clinics allows students to practise communication skills, assess patients, and understand management planning. These environments highlight the importance of teamwork and collaboration across specialties and professions, reinforcing the multidisciplinary nature of surgical care.

Finally, students are encouraged to engage in academic and quality improvement activities during their placements. Participation in audits or quality improvement projects develops practical skills in data collection, analysis, and implementation of change, while contributing meaningfully to patient care and clinical governance. Such experiences also strengthen a student's portfolio and demonstrate commitment to the specialty.

By approaching surgical placements with curiosity and enthusiasm, students can transform these experiences into a strong foundation for future training. Each placement offers not only an opportunity to acquire skills and knowledge but also a chance to reflect and take confident steps towards a career in surgery.

SURGICAL RECORD-KEEPING: eLOGBOOK

Students are strongly encouraged to begin maintaining a record of the operations and procedures they have been involved in, as this will be invaluable at later stages when applying for core or higher specialty training. This is most commonly achieved through the surgical eLogbook, an online platform that documents operative experience across a range of levels, from observation and assisting to performing procedures.

Registration for the eLogbook is free, and entering cases is a straightforward process. The patient details required for an eLogbook entry typically include patient identifiers, date of birth, the procedure performed, the supervising consultant, and the level of supervision, with the option to add further operative details if desired.

At this early stage, it is advisable to record all clinical experiences, including those undertaken in an observational capacity. Surgical training is inherently experiential, and maintaining a comprehensive and accurate log of procedures encountered demonstrates engagement and initiative in future applications. Additionally, the eLogbook serves as a useful personal record, helping students recall and reflect on their experiences during surgical placements when completing reflections or preparing future applications.

KEY GENERAL SURGICAL OPERATIONS

Within general surgery, a wide range of operations and clinical presentations can be observed which vary in complexity. These may be encountered during the acute general surgical take or while assisting with elective procedures. Cases performed on an emergency operating list may have an increased acuity in comparison to a planned elective list. The breadth of cases can seem overwhelming, and an exhaustive list of all general surgical operations is beyond the scope of this book. However, the following is a brief overview of some of the most commonly performed operations in general surgery. Broadly speaking, these operations may be carried out using an open technique (via direct access through the skin), a laparoscopic (minimally invasive or 'keyhole') approach using ports and a camera, using robotic-assisted technology, or a combination of the above techniques.

Hernia repair

- This involves repairing openings or defects in the abdominal wall through which tissues may protrude. Examples of hernia subtypes include inguinal, femoral, paraumbilical, epigastric, and incisional. Hernia surgery may be performed in the elective or emergency setting.

Cholecystectomy

- This is the operation for removal of the gallbladder, most commonly for symptomatic gallstones. Cholecystectomy surgery is commonly performed laparoscopically, and it may be undertaken in the elective or emergency setting.

Skin/subcutaneous lesion excision

- This involves the removal of a simple skin lesion such as an epidermal cyst, or a subcutaneous lesion such as a lipoma. This is typically performed under local anaesthesia.

Bowel resection

- This involves the partial removal of the small or large bowel for benign or malignant conditions. Bowel resection may be performed in the elective or emergency setting, through open or minimally invasive approaches, and is typically followed by the creation of an anastomosis (a join between the residual portions of the bowel to maintain continuity) or a stoma (bringing out the proximal end of the residual bowel to the abdominal wall to divert the gastrointestinal contents away from the rest of the gastrointestinal tract and into a bag).

Appendicectomy

- This involves the removal of the appendix.
- It is commonly undertaken laparoscopically in the emergency setting for acute appendicitis, or occasionally in the elective setting as 'interval' appendicectomy.

Incision and drainage

- This is an operation which involves releasing pus from an abscess from anywhere on the body. It can be done under local or general anaesthesia.

Laparotomy

- This is a major operation that involves opening the abdomen to treat a variety of emergent or elective conditions. It is typically undertaken through a vertical incision along the midline of the abdominal wall.

Haemorrhoidectomy

- This involves excision of haemorrhoids or "piles" which are dilated and displaced anal cushions that cause symptoms.

Mastectomy/lumpectomy

- This involves the removal of breast tissue (whole or a portion), typically for the treatment of cancer or sometimes benign conditions.

Thyroidectomy

- This involves the partial or total removal of the thyroid gland for benign or malignant conditions.

Splenectomy

- This involves the removal of the spleen due to trauma or benign or malignant haematological disorders.

Other types of surgical procedures may include more specialised operations such as transplant operations (kidney, pancreas, liver), oesophagectomy, fundoplication (anti-reflux surgery), bariatric surgery (metabolic weight-loss surgery), anterior resection (resection of the rectum), and many more within the various general surgical subspecialties. Where possible, reviewing the relevant anatomy, indications, and surgical steps in advance is strongly recommended to optimise learning and enhance intra-operative understanding.

Selecting medical electives

Electives, whether completed locally or abroad, can be guided by a medical student's area of interest. Surgical electives may be taken locally within or outside one's home institution, or abroad. Depending on the country and its available resources, students may encounter a range of practices and procedures. Witnessing alternative surgical practices in different institutions provides a global perspective and framework within surgical practice.

Success in securing a surgical elective often depends on planning and early application. Applying for an elective requires early insight and preparation because these applications must be undertaken months in advance. Having a good idea of what one would like to accomplish and discussing with senior students may be helpful to gain a good perspective. These placements can be highly competitive, especially those that offer funding, so careful planning is crucial. Fortunately, many universities and external organisations offer grants to help support these enriching educational experiences.

MEDICAL INTERCALATION

Aspiring surgeons are often encouraged to engage with academia at an early stage in their careers, and intercalation during the undergraduate years provides a meaningful opportunity to do so. Intercalation typically involves taking a compulsory or optional year out of the standard medical curriculum, depending on the medical school, to pursue an additional degree alongside medicine. This period offers valuable time for reflection, academic growth, and exploration of interests beyond the core medical course.

Intercalated degrees may be medically themed, such as surgical sciences or anatomy, allowing students to deepen their understanding of relevant subjects and develop foundational knowledge. There are also non-medical intercalated degrees in management, education, or global health, which are increasingly popular and offer transferable skills in leadership and innovation which are highly applicable to surgical practice.

For many students, intercalation sometimes serves as a gateway to academic medicine. It often provides early exposure to research through a dissertation or structured research project, helping students develop critical appraisal skills and an appreciation for evidence-based practice. This experience can open doors to future research opportunities and may strengthen applications later in training.

It is important to recognise that intercalation is not mandatory and may not be the right choice for everyone. When chosen thoughtfully, an intercalated year can be both professionally enriching and personally rewarding, offering space to reflect on one's aspirations while developing skills that will support future medical and surgical practice.

Research activities

Research plays a vital role in advancing healthcare by generating new insights into clinical practice and systems of care. For medical students, engaging in research can also serve as a meaningful way to deepen interest in surgery or other specialties, and such involvement is highly regarded in career progression. The intercalation year provides an invaluable opportunity to undertake research.

Research typically begins with a clinical or scientific question. Practically, a student may reach out to a supervisor working in a field of interest and be assigned a role within the research team. This role may range from data collection and analysis to scientific writing, with opportunities to present findings at conferences or contribute to publications.

Importantly, students should not feel pressured to undertake research solely in general surgery or their anticipated specialty. At this nascent stage in one's career, all research experience is valuable, even in unrelated fields. Pursuing a project in an area one is genuinely interested in is advisable since balancing research with medical school demands can be challenging. Passion for the subject often provides the motivation needed to see a project through to completion.

To get started, students are encouraged to approach lecturers or clinicians who may be involved in ongoing projects. Demonstrating enthusiasm and a willingness to contribute can open doors to research opportunities. In parallel, gaining a foundational understanding of research principles, particularly within medical and surgical contexts, will be beneficial when developing a research question and committing to a project. Alternatively, collaborative projects performed in conjunction with national or international surgical societies can be a useful introduction to research.

Ultimately, all research experience is worthwhile, regardless of the final output. Each project contributes to the development of critical thinking, collaboration, and communication skills, and helps build a research portfolio that may support future academic or clinical applications.

Examples of common research projects may include:

1. Systematic reviews: A systematic review collects all available literature and information on a research question in a structured format, and provides a qualitative or quantitative synthesis of available data. This can be a good starting project for students to pursue, as this can be done in one's own time to increase knowledge surrounding a research topic, and to improve key skills such as critical appraisal and literature searching.
2. Randomised controlled trials: Randomised controlled trials (RCTs) are prospective studies that measure the effectiveness of a new intervention or treatment in a structured manner. Students may get involved through supporting recruitment in an RCT, helping design proposals and ethical approvals, or through participation in patient-public involvement via surveys.
3. Observational study: These look at existing patient data and demographics through medical charts, records, databases to analyse past events, outcomes or correlations. These are often interesting to get involved in during surgical placements and can improve skills with statistical analysis and data handling.
4. Case reports or case series: Case reports are a narrative of a single patient or several patients with interesting conditions or atypical presentations which detail history, examination, diagnosis, treatment, and outcome. This is often an amenable project to get involved with as a student and provides a good introduction to scientific writing.

AUDITS AND QUALITY IMPROVEMENT PROJECTS (QIPS)

Clinical audit is a core element of clinical governance, involving the systematic comparison of current clinical practice against established best practice standards with the goal of enhancing patient care and service delivery. Improvements identified through audit may be implemented via QIPs, which are increasingly recognised as valuable contributions to healthcare systems. These projects often follow a P-D-S-A cycle (Plan-Do-Study-Act), a structured process that seeks to improve upon an existing pathway to an agreed standard.

Medical students are strongly encouraged to engage in clinical audit and quality improvement initiatives, as these experiences can significantly enrich their professional development and strengthen their portfolios. These projects may be difficult to start alone, so finding a mentor in a senior colleague or surgeon can provide a useful clinical perspective to understand what may be needed to improve a healthcare process or delivery of a service.

However, it is important to balance these activities with the demands of medical school. Taking on a manageable project that can be seen through to completion is often more beneficial than attempting to juggle multiple commitments without achieving meaningful outcomes. A well-executed, high-quality project with tangible results often holds more value than several incomplete or superficial efforts. These QIPs can be presented locally or at national or international conferences as posters or oral presentations, and provide a useful perspective for future practice.

SUPPLEMENTARY OPPORTUNITIES AND ACTIVITIES FOR PROFESSIONAL DEVELOPMENT

Surgical societies and related interest groups

Demonstrating commitment to a surgical specialty and exploring one's interest in surgery can be effectively achieved through active participation or leadership within surgical societies at the university or regional and national level. Involvement in organisations such as the Association of Surgeons in Training (ASiT), the Royal College of Surgeons of England (RCSEng), and similar bodies provides valuable opportunities for professional development, including access to educational events, networking platforms, and a wide range of learning resources.

Taking on leadership roles in committees within these societies can be particularly rewarding, offering experiences that extend beyond the development of leadership skills alone. Such positions allow students to engage with a broader community of aspiring surgeons, foster collaboration, and build professional networks that may prove beneficial throughout their careers.

Courses and conferences aimed at students

Attending or participating in surgical conferences at the university or national and international levels offers significant benefits for aspiring surgeons. There are a range of conferences that encourage medical student participation. These events provide exposure to the latest developments and innovations in general surgery, offering a unique opportunity for academic enrichment through accredited sessions and expert-led discussions. Presenting research, whether in the form of a poster, oral, or video presentation, not only enhances personal and professional development but also strengthens one's research portfolio. Such experiences foster critical thinking, improve communication skills, and may open doors to future academic opportunities within the surgical field.

The growing emphasis on simulation-based education and technical skill development has led to the introduction of structured surgical courses within the undergraduate curriculum. Notable examples include the RCS Surgical Skills for Students (SSS) course and the Introduction to Vascular Surgery course by the Rouleaux Club, among others. These initiatives offer students early access to core surgical techniques, enhance confidence in clinical settings, and support informed career decision-making.

Working in anatomy laboratories

Medical students with an interest in a surgical career may have the opportunity to gain early clinical exposure through internships in university anatomy laboratories. These experiences provide valuable hands-on learning and a deeper understanding of surgical anatomy, an essential foundation for future surgical training.

Medical secretarial work

There may be opportunities to work with a senior consultant or a team of medical professionals in a medical secretarial capacity. These roles are typically offered on an ad-hoc or part-time basis. As well as providing practical exposure to medical terminology and clinical documentation, offering beneficial learning experiences, they can serve as a valuable source of supplementary income.

Finding a mentor – guidance for a career

Mentorship has been consistently linked to enhanced career development, increased motivation, and greater success in achieving professional goals, particularly within specialised fields. For medical students aspiring to pursue a career in surgery, the guidance of an experienced surgical mentor can be especially valuable. A mentor can provide informed career advice, facilitate reflective learning, and offer insight into the day-to-day realities of the surgical profession.

Identifying and establishing a mentoring relationship, however, can be a daunting process. Medical students are encouraged to actively engage with surgeons across all levels of training during clinical placements, as well as to seek guidance from academic tutors and faculty members.

Additional mentorship opportunities may also be available through surgical societies, professional networks, or formal institutional mentoring programmes. Taking the initiative to connect with potential mentors can significantly enrich the educational experience and support informed career decision-making.

BALANCING YOUR PERSPECTIVE

Maintaining balance is an essential, and often challenging, part of navigating medical school. While an early interest in surgery can be a powerful source of motivation and purpose, it is worth taking time to reflect on the broader goal of medical training: becoming a competent, compassionate, and well-rounded doctor. This requires thoughtful engagement with all aspects of the curriculum, not solely those aligned with a future surgical ambition.

Medical school demands the careful balancing of academic work, clinical placements, and assessments, alongside personal well-being. Learning to manage time and energy effectively is a gradual process, and one that benefits from regular reflection. Investing in areas beyond immediate interests not only strengthens clinical foundations, but also deepens understanding of how different specialties intersect in patient care.

In the early years of training, keeping an open and flexible mindset can be particularly valuable. Exposure to a wide range of clinical environments often reshapes perspectives, and it is not uncommon for career aspirations to evolve with experience. While enthusiasm for surgery is positive, becoming too fixed on a single outcome too early may limit opportunities for growth and discovery.

Approaching career planning with a sense of curiosity rather than certainty, i.e. "planning in pencil" rather than ink allows space for change. Adaptability, openness, and self-awareness are qualities that develop over time and underpin both professional fulfilment and resilience. Reflecting regularly on your experiences can help ensure that your journey through medical school remains balanced, purposeful, and aligned with your developing values.

BIBLIOGRAPHY

Acquaah F, Goldsmith T, McNally S. How to make the most of your surgical placement. British Medical Journal. 2017 Sep 5, 358;j3718.

ACS. So you want to be a surgeon [Internet]. ACS. Available from: https://www.facs.org/for-medical-professionals/education/programs/so-you-want-to-be-a-surgeon/

BMJ. The complete guide to becoming a general surgeon [Internet]. *BMJ Careers*. 2023. Available from: https://www.bmj.com/careers/article/the-complete-guide-to-becoming-a-general-surgeon-

Gera R. A realistic guide to surgical rotations – A realistic guide to medical school [Internet]. Ucl.ac.uk. 2020 [cited 2024 Nov 12]. Available from: https://reflect.ucl.ac.uk/argtm/2020/11/12/a-realistic-guide-to-surgical-rotations/

Jamadar·Blog T. Making the most of your clinical placements | Geeky medics [Internet]. 2019. Available from: https://geekymedics.com/making-the-most-of-your-clinical-placements/

Nadarajah S. Clinical placement [Internet]. The British Medical Association is the trade union and professional body for doctors in the UK. 2024. Available from: https://www.bma.org.uk/advice-and-support/studying-medicine/support-at-medical-school/clinical-placement

RCS Edinburgh. The path from school to surgery | RCSEd [Internet]. Rcsed.ac.uk. 2024 [cited 2024 Nov 12]. Available from: https://www.rcsed.ac.uk/professional-support-development-resources/career-support/career-advice-for-school-pupils/the-path-from-school-to-surgery

RCS Edinburgh. How can I get ahead? [Internet]. The Royal College of Surgeons of Edinburgh. Available from: https://www.rcsed.ac.uk/professional-support-development-resources/career-support/career-advice-for-medical-students/how-can-i-get-ahead

RCS England. Applying to medical school [Internet]. Royal College of Surgeons. Available from: https://www.rcseng.ac.uk/careers-in-surgery/careers-support/applying-to-medical-school/

RCS England. Improving your chances of entering surgical training [Internet]. Royal College of Surgeons. Available from: https://www.rcseng.ac.uk/careers-in-surgery/medical-students/improving-your-chances-of-entering-surgical-training/

RCS England. Students – Royal college of surgeons [Internet]. Royal College of Surgeons. 2024. Available from: https://www.rcseng.ac.uk/careers-in-surgery/medical-students/

RCS England. Surgery entry requirements and training [Internet]. Royal College of Surgeons. Available from: https://www.rcseng.ac.uk/careers-in-surgery/careers-support/what-is-surgery-like-as-a-career/entry-requirements-and-training/

3

The early years: Foundation training

INTRODUCTION

Foundation training is a structured, two-year postgraduate medical training programme that serves as a critical transition between medical school and speciality training. During this period, newly qualified doctors undertake a series of clinical rotations across a range of specialties. The exact split of each rotation differs depending on the job and deanery. These rotations which take place during Foundation Year 1 (FY1) and Foundation Year 2 (FY2) are carefully supervised and designed to provide trainees with broad clinical exposure, enabling them to develop the foundational skills, knowledge, and professional behaviours necessary to function effectively as foundation doctors.

The programme aims to support the transition from the academic environment of medical school to the practical and often demanding responsibilities of clinical practice. Through exposure to a variety of clinical settings and patient populations, foundation trainees gain invaluable experience in clinical assessment, decision-making, and multidisciplinary teamwork, while progressively developing autonomy under supervision. This generalist period of a doctor's initial training is designed for preparation for the next stages of practice within a subspecialty.

The transition from medical student to foundation doctor can be both challenging and transformative, marking a period of significant personal and professional development. Working as a foundation doctor provides a unique opportunity to gain practical experience in both

DOI: 10.1201/9781003537663-3

surgical and non-surgical specialties. Through activities such as assessing acutely unwell patients, participating in clinical decision-making, and learning to manage competing demands, foundation doctors begin to shape their approach to medical practice, skills that will influence their careers long-term.

For those considering a career in surgery, foundation training serves as an important phase to explore the specialty in greater depth, affirm career intentions, and build relevant experience prior to applying for Core Surgical Training (CST). These two years are also crucial for maintaining a balanced perspective, as doctors adapt to the realities of clinical practice while developing their professional identity.

This chapter outlines the opportunities available during foundation training to begin building a competitive surgical portfolio and to prepare effectively for CST applications.

FOUNDATION DOCTORS AND THE TRADITIONAL HOUSE OFFICER MODEL

The UK postgraduate medical training system has evolved from the traditional house officer model to the current Foundation Programme, consisting of FY1 and FY2. While these roles are historically linked, they differ formally in structure. The traditional house officer role, which predated the Foundation Programme, included pre-registration house officers (PRHO) and senior house officers (SHOs). Training was often service led with variable supervision and progression depended largely on local practice rather than a nationally defined curriculum.

FY1 has replaced the PRHO role. It marks the transition from medical student to practicing doctor, with a focus on developing core clinical skills under close supervision. Completion of FY1 is required for full registration with the General Medical Council. FY2 corresponds to the early stage of the former SHO grade. FY2 doctors assume greater responsibility compared to FY1 doctors and contribute more actively to clinical decision-making in preparation for entry into specialty or core training programmes.

This shift reflects a move towards a more structured, competency-based approach to postgraduate medical education, with clearer expectations and improved continuity of training (Figure 3.1).

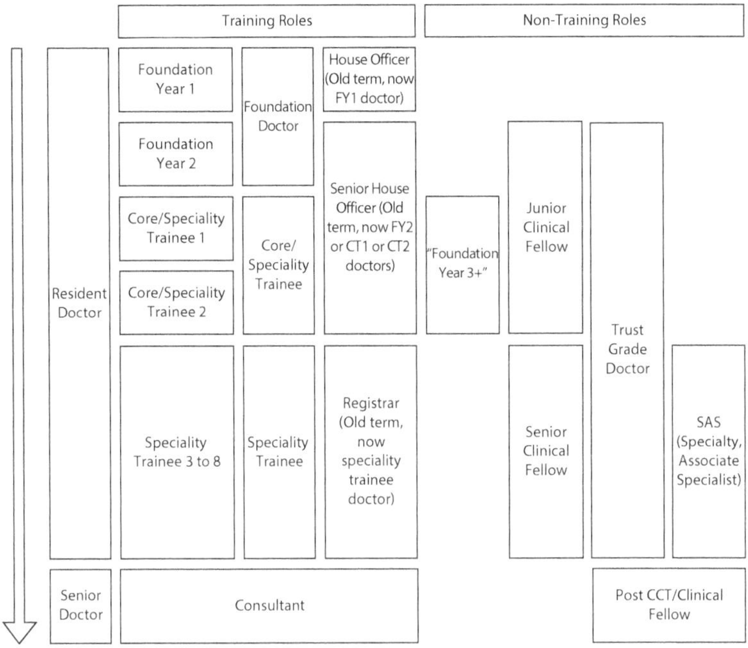

Figure 3.1 Roles of resident doctor grades in the UK and the different terms used to describe them.

ROLES AND RESPONSIBILITIES OF FOUNDATION DOCTORS

While the majority of foundation programmes consist of three four-month rotations, alternative structures such as two six-month or four three-month placements may also be offered, depending on the training scheme. The roles and responsibilities of foundation doctors are varied and dynamic, often differing significantly between individual placements and specialties. As such, it is important for trainees to familiarise themselves early with the expectations specific to each rotation. Ahead of starting a rotation, trainees are encouraged to get in contact with doctors they will be taking over from to understand what the roles and responsibilities of the job. Clear communication with supervisors and senior colleagues at the outset of a placement can help ensure that responsibilities are understood and that trainees are appropriately integrated into the clinical team. With any medical or surgical rotation, one may find it difficult to find their feet in a new environment. Remember that it is expected of foundation doctors to ask if they are unsure of a decision or a process, and that seniors are often willing to help.

Across all rotations, a core component of the foundation doctor's role is the provision of inpatient care. This includes tasks such as reviewing patients on ward rounds, initiating and following up on investigations, prescribing under supervision, communicating with patients and their families, and coordinating care with the wider multidisciplinary team through referrals and discussions. Foundation doctors serve as a key point of contact for patients on the ward and play a crucial role in maintaining continuity of care. The foundation doctor is also often the first point of contact for nursing staff and administrative staff, receiving input from different members of the multidisciplinary team (MDT) regarding the care of their patients.

In surgical placements, the scope of responsibilities often expands beyond the ward environment. Foundation trainees will be expected to assist in the operating theatre, attend surgical outpatient clinics, and participate in pre- and post-operative care. The extent of involvement in these activities may depend on the trainee's level of experience, the needs of the department, and local rota arrangements. Nonetheless, such exposure offers valuable insight into surgical workflows and patient pathways and provides opportunities to develop procedural and decision-making skills. Much like placements in medical school, some sub-specialist surgical rotations may provide a more supernumerary experience for foundation doctors. This is often a good opportunity to immerse oneself in assisting in theatres and observing outpatient clinics without regular ward commitments.

Out-of-hours work, including evening, overnight, and weekend shifts, is another essential aspect of foundation training. During these periods, foundation doctors may be responsible for clerking new admissions from the emergency department, reviewing unwell patients on the wards, and supporting the acute medical or surgical take. In particular, participating in the acute surgical take offers a unique opportunity to gain experience in the assessment and initial management of common surgical presentations and to observe the decision-making processes involved in emergency surgery. Foundation doctors may also be expected to receive surgical referrals from other clinical teams under the supervision of a senior doctor.

In addition to clinical duties, foundation doctors are often expected to contribute to the administrative and governance aspects of patient care. This may include preparing for and attending MDT meetings, contributing to morbidity and mortality (M&M) reviews, or participating in clinical governance and quality improvement initiatives. Engaging with these activities not only enhances a trainee's understanding of the wider healthcare system but also supports the development of skills in leadership, communication, and clinical audit competencies that are essential for progression in any medical or surgical specialty.

Overall, the Foundation Programme is designed to provide a broad and balanced experience that equips resident doctors with the skills and professionalism required for the next stage of training. Although each specific placement may differ, understanding and fulfilling the roles expected in each placement is key to maximising learning and delivering safe and effective patient care. There is much to gain from all placements regardless of speciality, and these years are formative to a doctor's future practice.

THE FOUNDATION PROGRAMME CURRICULUM AND ASSESSMENTS

The Foundation Programme curriculum outlines the core learning objectives and competencies that foundation doctors are expected to achieve in order to support their educational and professional development. These "Foundation Professional Capabilities" (FPCs) reflect key components of the clinical or professional aspect of clinical practice. It encompasses a broad range of domains beyond traditional clinical skills, including communication and consultation, reflective practice, and effective teamwork. Underpinning these FPCs are expectations of a doctor's commitment to regular reflection, lifelong learning, and professionalism.

Foundation doctors are required to demonstrate competence across these domains by actively engaging with the curriculum. Familiarity with the curriculum is essential, and trainees are encouraged to use it as a framework to guide their day-to-day learning and long-term progression.

Progression in foundation training is structured and awards certificates at each year's completion. After FY1 is completed with a satisfactory Annual Review of Competence Progression (ARCP) outcome, an award of the Foundation Year 1 Certificate of Completion (F1CC), GMC Certificate of Experience and progression to FY 2 is recommended. After satisfactory ARCP and completion of the second Foundation Year, award of the Foundation Programme Certificate of Completion (FPCC) is made, which allows trainees to enter core or specialty training programmes. Therefore, it is of paramount importance to maintain good records and evidence to support one's progression.

To support this process, an electronic portfolio system called Horus is used to document learning, capture evidence of progress, and facilitate structured reflection. The e-portfolio serves as a central repository for assessments, feedback, and personal development activities, and is a key tool in preparing for the ARCP. Horus is the primary system used in England, and the specific platform may vary in Scotland, Wales, and Ireland. All these platforms aim to fulfil a similar role in the assessment of resident doctors and their progression.

Workplace-Based Assessments (WBAs) form an integral part of the assessment framework. These are intended to provide formative, structured feedback on a trainee's performance in real clinical settings, helping to identify learning needs and guide development. Specific numbers of each WBA may be established by each local trust

Common WBAs include:

- *Case-Based Discussions (CBD)*: Structured discussion of a clinical case that a foundation doctor has managed or observed. This reflects a foundation doctor's ability to use clinical information and develop their clinical reasoning.
- *Mini-Clinical Evaluation Exercises (Mini-CEX)*: An observed clinical encounter of a foundation doctor's clinical evaluation of a patient which may include history, examination, and relevant communications with patients and their families.
- *Direct Observation of Procedural Skills (DOPS)*: Practical procedures such as venepuncture, catheterisation, and suturing which is witnessed by a senior assessor.

In addition to WBAs, foundation doctors are also assessed through Multisource Feedback (MSF), also referred to as Team Assessment of Behaviour (TAB), which gathers insights into a trainee's professional conduct from a broad range of colleagues, including medical staff, allied health professionals, and, where applicable, patients. Reflective practice is also a key component of the curriculum. Trainees are expected to make regular, thoughtful entries that demonstrate critical reflection on clinical experiences, ethical challenges, and professional growth. These reflections can be done individually or in collaboration with other colleagues.

There are also mandatory courses such as Advanced Life Support (ALS) which must be completed during foundation training. There is an expectation that foundation doctors attend a specific number of hours of teaching provided by the local trust or deanery, which may occur on a weekly or monthly basis depending on local policies. In addition to this, foundation doctors may be expected to fulfil a "Developing the Clinical Teacher" requirement which entails provision of a teaching session and associated reflections. In addition, completion of administrative forms such as Form R is required for a successful ARCP.

During both surgical and non-surgical placements, it is generally recommended that trainees go beyond the minimum required number of WBAs. Actively seeking out assessments, requesting timely and specific feedback, and engaging in meaningful reflection can significantly enhance learning and support ongoing professional development. This can be supported by fostering a good relationship with senior colleagues and consultants, and often resident doctors may find useful and synchronous feedback to their WBAs when asked. It is often high-quality WBAs that are useful for a foundation doctor's learning. Trainees are encouraged to remember that these are distinct learning activities that support learning rather than checkbox exercises.

The following are a few important tips to ensuring that your portfolio remains up-to-date and high quality.

1. Ensure you are proactive in seeking WBAs: foundation doctors are expected to be self-driven and motivated, and to seek opportunities when available to discuss cases or perform clinical skills. This often means finding an amenable senior colleague to observe and provide feedback. Sending tickets immediately or soon after an encounter ensures the feedback is fresh in a supervisor's mind and increases the likelihood that the WBA is signed off.
2. Stay organised and update your e-portfolio regularly, checking this against your personal development plan for a particular rotation: Keeping regular reminders to update one's portfolio monthly can be a useful exercise. If you are finding it difficult to go to teaching or to gain sufficient WBAs or eLogbook experience, it may be useful to escalate to one's educational supervisor or clinical supervisor who may be able to assist. Maintain a high-quality, well-rounded portfolio that includes evidence of projects (audits, QiPs, research) and additional activities such as leadership, management and teaching as these feature in the scoring system for core training applications.

SURGICAL ELOGBOOK: BEYOND THE PORTFOLIO

It is important to note that much like medical school, the maintenance of accurate records of operations that a foundation doctor has observed or participated in is vital for future applications to core surgical or higher speciality training. There is an expectation of progression from medical school, a transition from observation into assisting or even performing procedures is expected for CST applications. There is an expected number of 40 procedures that a foundation doctor can assist in, which can provide a boost for their portfolio, although it is important to strive for as much experience as possible beyond this number.

Selecting foundation placements: An essential bridge to speciality training

The selection and allocation processes for foundation training posts are currently undergoing significant reforms. At the time of writing this book, the allocation system was evolving from a model incorporating decile rankings and situational judgement test (SJT) scores towards a more randomised allocation approach. Given that this system is subject to ongoing change, applicants are strongly advised to consult the most current guidance and updates published by Health Education England (HEE) and the national application platform, Oriel. Staying informed about these changes is essential for making well-informed application decisions.

For those aspiring to pursue a career in surgery, it is advisable to prioritise foundation placements that include a greater proportion of surgical rotations. Early exposure to surgical specialties during foundation training provides valuable opportunities to develop technical skills, understand the workflow within surgical teams, and gain insight into the demands and rewards of surgical practice.

When selecting foundation training placements, prospective trainees should conduct research regarding the various hospital trusts and training environments. In reality, there is considerable variability between hospitals in terms of teaching quality, clinical workload, support structures, and overall trainee experience. Engaging with current or past foundation doctors at prospective sites can offer invaluable, practical insights that complement official programme descriptions. This due diligence can aid in making strategic choices that align with individual career goals and personal circumstances.

SURGICAL ROTATIONS WITHIN FOUNDATION TRAINING

Gaining firsthand experience across various surgical specialties during foundation training is invaluable in the early stages of a medical career. The skills acquired in one surgical subspecialty are often transferable and applicable to others, providing a broad clinical foundation. Exposure to diverse surgical fields not only reinforces your interest in pursuing a career in surgery but also assists in refining your choice of speciality.

Foundation training, particularly within busy surgical wards, can be both mentally and physically demanding. Effective organisation and time management are crucial skills that develop with experience and are essential for managing the workload. Support is readily available from clinical and educational supervisors, postgraduate groups, and colleagues, and trainees are encouraged to seek guidance whenever needed. Despite the challenges, do not allow these demands to deter you from engaging fully with theatre sessions, clinics, and other surgical environments.

To optimise learning during surgical rotations, it is beneficial to set clear personal objectives. These may include maintaining a surgical logbook, actively participating in theatre by scrubbing in to assist with operations, clerking surgical patients to observe a broad spectrum of surgical conditions, or contributing to research and audit projects. Assisting in theatres is likely to be the first step as a foundation doctor, and there are several tips to becoming an excellent assistant. It is vital to anticipate a surgeon's needs and develop skills such as suturing and haemostasis. In addition, learning to perform the World Health Organization Surgical Safety Checklist and sign outs are useful skills to develop. When in the operating theatre, introducing oneself to the surgeon and wider team, including the anaesthetic doctors, scrub nurses and theatre practitioners, is often the first step. One may find it beneficial to attend courses such as Basic Surgical Skills (BSS) during foundation training prior to starting a surgical placement, which can provide a useful baseline knowledge of practical surgery and increase confidence in operating theatres.

Maximising theatre opportunities is particularly important regardless of the surgical specialty. The operating theatre is an unparalleled learning environment where trainees can develop practical skills such as suturing and assisting. Equally valuable are the interpersonal skills honed in this setting, including effective communication, professionalism, and adaptability. While some foundation doctors may have designated theatre days, others can demonstrate their enthusiasm by proactively engaging with consultants or registrars. It is essential to prioritise and complete all clinical responsibilities before participating in theatre sessions to support the wider clinical team effectively. Additional valuable experiences include shadowing senior surgical colleagues during acute on-call shifts or outpatient clinics, which offer insight into the roles and responsibilities of higher surgical trainees.

When applying for core and higher surgical training, demonstrating a consistent and genuine commitment to the specialty is highly regarded. Actively engaging in the opportunities outlined earlier not only enriches your foundation training experience but also strengthens your surgical portfolio and supports your long-term career development.

NON-SURGICAL ROTATIONS

All foundation trainees will rotate through a range of medical and community-based specialties as part of their training. While these placements may not directly align with surgical practice, they provide essential clinical experience and should not be undervalued by those aspiring for a career in surgery.

Non-surgical rotations offer a critical foundation in the principles of general medical care, which is vital for managing acute presentations in any clinical setting, including surgical wards. These placements help develop core competencies such as diagnostic reasoning, clinical decision-making, and management of increasingly complex and co-morbid patient populations. Furthermore, they foster independence, improve communication across multidisciplinary teams, and strengthen the ability to manage patients holistically.

For surgical aspirants, the skills acquired during medical and community-based placements are highly transferable and will serve as a strong foundation for future surgical training. Engaging fully in all rotations, regardless of specialty, demonstrates professionalism and a commitment to comprehensive clinical development.

It is essential not to overlook the learning opportunities in non-surgical placements. Embracing the breadth of the Foundation Programme will ultimately enhance both clinical competence and confidence, supporting success in future surgical training and beyond.

TASTER WEEKS

Taster weeks provide exposure to specialties that a foundation trainee may not have the opportunity to experience during their scheduled rotations. These placements offer a unique opportunity to gain deeper insights into a particular field of interest, helping to inform future career decisions and demonstrate commitment to a chosen specialty. Taster weeks are often taken within a deanery or healthcare trust, and special permission must be sought to take a taster week outside one's locality.

Organising a taster week requires careful planning and coordination. Trainees should liaise with their clinical supervisor and rota coordinator to arrange study leave at a convenient time. It is also necessary to contact consultants or heads of department, ideally those with whom the trainee has a professional interest or prior connection, via email or formal letter to request their support in facilitating the placement. There may be frameworks in place which allow doctors to contact consultants for permission to attend taster weeks in some deaneries; however, these are often arranged on an ad hoc basis. In some instances, approval may also be required from the trainee's current educational or clinical supervisor.

Taster weeks typically range from one to five consecutive days and can be structured to include clinical shadowing, attendance at departmental meetings, participation in teaching sessions, and other relevant specialty-specific activities. When well-planned, these experiences are often highly informative and rewarding. Although it may be daunting to start at a different department, it is important to note that this taster is an observational experience to gain insight into a speciality, and not a work placement as such.

Upon completion of the taster, it is advisable to obtain formal documentation or a letter from the supervising consultant confirming attendance and outlining the activities undertaken. This serves as useful evidence for future training applications and contributes to a portfolio demonstrating early career exploration and commitment.

RECOMMENDED COURSES, CONFERENCES, AND WORKSHOPS

Foundation trainees are strongly encouraged to engage in relevant conferences, courses, and workshops as part of their ongoing professional development. Prestigious national organisations such as the Royal College of Surgeons (RCS), Royal College of Physicians (RCP), Royal Society of Medicine (RSM), and HEE regularly host high-quality educational events tailored to early career doctors.

In addition, surgical specialty groups including the Association of Surgeons in Training (ASiT), Cooper's club (for hernia enthusiasts) and the Dukes' Club (for colorectal trainees) actively welcome participation from foundation doctors, offering valuable opportunities to present work, network with peers, and gain insight into specialty training pathways. There are often awards and prizes for research projects, essays or travel grants which can provide a boost for one's portfolio in future applications.

To stay organised and make the most of these opportunities, consider creating a year-long calendar of specialty-specific events, including key deadlines for registration and abstract submissions. Set aside time each month to review newly announced events and calls for abstracts to ensure you remain informed and can plan your involvement effectively.

STAYING COMPETITIVE AND DEMONSTRATING COMMITMENT TO SPECIALTY

Standing out in surgical training applications requires more than clinical competence; it demands a well-rounded, proactive approach to professional development. Building a strong portfolio through research, teaching, leadership, and quality improvement initiatives not only enhances your application but also demonstrates genuine commitment to your chosen specialty.

Engaging in research alongside clinical responsibilities can be demanding, yet it is an excellent way to show intellectual curiosity and dedication. Get involved in academic projects, submit essays for national prizes, and present your work at conferences whenever possible. Similarly, audits and quality improvement (QI) projects remain essential components of a robust application. Rather than focusing on the number of audits completed, selection panels are more interested in whether you've closed the audit loop and demonstrated leadership in driving change. Consider projects on common topics and practical areas such as clerking proformas, analgesia, antibiotic stewardship, or Intravenous fluid prescribing. Don't hesitate to ask your seniors for ideas or support – they may have more clinical insight into high yield audits which can promote change where needed.

Teaching and volunteering also play a vital role in showcasing your communication, leadership, and mentoring skills. Whether you're delivering formal teaching sessions, mentoring junior colleagues, or supporting student surgical societies, these experiences reflect a dedication to service and professional growth. It is important to gain formal feedback either online or written for teaching sessions as this can be used as evidence in applications of the teaching activity.

Leadership experience is increasingly valued in specialty applications. Opportunities may include helping to develop local departmental guidelines, contributing to induction packs for new doctors, or proposing solutions to improve existing clinical processes. Formal roles such as Foundation Year representative, Doctor's Mess President, or membership in hospital or national committees (e.g. ASiT Foundation Representatives) can be demanding, but they provide excellent platforms to influence change and develop essential skills.

For those seeking structured development, consider enrolling in recognised leadership programmes such as those offered by the Healthcare Leadership Academy or the Faculty of Medical Leadership and Management (FMLM). The NHS Edward Jenner programme is a free introduction to healthcare leadership and can be attended in one's own time.

Finally, take advantage of careers fairs and specialty-specific events hosted by the Royal Colleges and the Royal Society of Medicine (RSM). These events offer valuable insight into the realities of surgical careers and allow you to connect with clinicians across specialties. Not only will this help confirm your motivation, but it also signals to selection panels that you have taken a thoughtful and informed approach to your career path, demonstrating both initiative and long-term commitment.

PREPARING FOR CORE SURGICAL TRAINING (CST) APPLICATIONS

The landscape of surgical training is continuously evolving, with frequent updates to curricula and recruitment processes. It is essential to familiarise yourself early with the most up-to-date person specification and application guidance available via HEE/NHS England's Specialty Recruitment website (http://specialtytraining.hee.nhs.uk/specialty-recruitment/). Regularly review these documents throughout your foundation years to identify any gaps in your portfolio and actively work to address them.

Whatever activities you undertake to demonstrate commitment to surgery, whether research, teaching, leadership, audits, or clinical experiences, it is crucial to maintain accurate records. Ensure all evidence, including certificates, sign-offs, and reflective entries, is well-organised and readily accessible. The application process can be time-pressured, and chasing missing documentation at the last minute can be stressful and potentially detrimental. It is recommended to start collating evidence months in advance prior to the application deadline. Examples of successful evidence may be found on the application website, or from previous successful applicants.

Your foundation years are a pivotal time to develop a competitive application. It's never too late to start, but showing that you've consistently engaged with learning opportunities, taken initiative, and maximised your time during these two years will significantly strengthen your application.

As you approach the CST application stage, always refer to the latest guidance provided by HEE and NHS England to ensure you are aligning with current expectations. With increasing competition across most surgical specialties, it is more important than ever to be proactive. For competition ratios, visit the HEE Specialty Recruitment (http://specialtytraining.hee.nhs.uk/specialty-recruitment/) page online. Seek out opportunities that enhance your portfolio and set you apart.

Ultimately, your career progression is your responsibility. The effort, time, and organisation you invest now will directly influence your future success in securing a place in surgical training.

TIME AFTER FOUNDATION TRAINING – THE "F3" YEAR AND BEYOND

Upon completing the two-year Foundation Programme, many doctors choose to take time out of formal training before entering specialty pathways. This has become an increasingly popular and accepted option, with many opting for an "F3 year", a term often extended to "F4" or beyond, depending on the duration of the break.

There are a variety of reasons doctors may choose to pause their training, including exploring different career options, gaining clinical experience in new environments, undertaking higher degrees such as a master's or PhD, or preparing for postgraduate membership exams. Whatever the motivation, this time can be an invaluable opportunity for personal and professional growth. The following are some of the common pathways taken after FY2.

Clinical posts and locum work

Many doctors take on clinical roles such as trust-grade positions or work as locum doctors. These posts allow flexibility, financial stability, and the chance to explore different specialties or hospitals. Availability varies by region, so early planning is advisable. There is increasing competition for these trust-grade posts, therefore, seeking opportunities in one's local department may be a good first lead before casting a wider net. These roles are often advertised internally or on the NHS Jobs website, and it is important to regularly check or set alerts for these jobs.

Teaching and leadership opportunities

Roles such as Clinical Teaching Fellow, Simulation Fellow, or Anatomy Demonstrator provide excellent opportunities to develop teaching skills while staying clinically involved. These posts may involve some level of clinical work in addition to teaching commitments, and are highly sought after. These posts often support exam preparation and may include the option to pursue a Postgraduate Certificate in Medical Education (PGCert), which adds further value to your Curriculum Vitae (CV). Involvement with the university and design of the medical school curriculum are also key advantages, providing insight into a potential future career in education and academics.

Working abroad

Practicing medicine in countries like Australia, New Zealand, or Singapore is a popular option for many UK-trained doctors. These placements offer exposure to new healthcare systems, diverse clinical experiences, and the opportunity to travel. Complete immersion in a new healthcare system can provide benefits and expand one's clinical practice whilst growing new connections. Some foundation doctors may even choose to remain in the countries they practice in for longer term training. Early preparation is key, as visa processes and registration requirements can take several months. These processes vary between countries, and it is important to be conscientious and check early for any visa or medical regulatory requirements.

Research, higher education, and courses

Some doctors pursue academic interests by enrolling in master's programmes, PhDs, or diplomas in areas aligned with their specialty ambitions. Research fellow posts are another excellent way to contribute to the academic field while demonstrating long-term commitment to a particular specialty. These can range between one to three years in duration and may also involve clinical commitments depending on the individual job. These research jobs provide an additional benefit of availing a doctor with opportunities to work on high-impact projects which can result in national or international presentations and publications to hone one's CV.

Taking time out of training is not a step back. It can be a strategic move towards a more informed, enriched, and confident entry into specialty training.

CONCLUSION

The Foundation Programme represents a pivotal moment in a young doctor's journey, marking the shift from the relative structure of medical school to the responsibilities and realities of clinical practice. It can feel overwhelming at times: the steep learning curve, the long hours, and the constant awareness that your decisions now carry real weight. Yet it is precisely within this intensity that the programme finds its value.

Over these two years, you are not simply learning how to manage patients or navigate hospital systems; you are beginning to shape the kind of doctor you will become. Each rotation offers lessons beyond the curriculum about teamwork, resilience, communication, and self-awareness. There will be moments of self-doubt but also moments of quiet pride when skills you once observed from the side lines become second nature in your own hands.

For those drawn towards surgery, the Foundation Programme is especially formative. It provides early exposure to the clinical environment of theatres and wards, but equally important, it introduces you to the discipline, perseverance, and reflective practice that underpin a surgical career. Embracing this period with openness and reflection allows it to become a meaningful chapter in your development as a doctor.

BIBLIOGRAPHY

Anon. Applying to Core Surgical Training (CST) [Internet]. *Mind The Bleep*. 2021 [cited 2024 Nov 12]. Available from: https://mindthebleep.com/applying-to-cst/

BMJ. A guide to the foundation programme for doctors [Internet]. *BMJ Careers*. Available from: https://www.bmj.com/careers/article/a-guide-to-the-foundation-programme-for-doctors

Health Education England. Core surgical training self assessment scoring guidance for candidates | Health Education England [Internet]. Health Education England | Medical Hub. 2024. Available from: https://medical.hee.nhs.uk/medical-training-recruitment/medical-specialty-training/surgery/core-surgery/core-surgical-training-self-assessment-scoring-guidance-for-candidates

Jamadar T. Making the Most of your Clinical Placements | Geeky Medics [Internet]. 2019. Available from: https://geekymedics.com/making-the-most-of-your-clinical-placements/

Nadarajah S. Clinical placement [Internet]. The British Medical Association is the trade union and professional body for doctors in the UK. Available from: https://www.bma.org.uk/advice-and-support/studying-medicine/support-at-medical-school/clinical-placement

NHS. Applying for foundation training [Internet]. *Health Careers*. 2015. Available from: https://www.healthcareers.nhs.uk/explore-roles/doctors/foundation-training/applying-foundation-training

NHS UK. Foundation training [Internet]. *Health Careers*. 2015. Available from: https://www.healthcareers.nhs.uk/explore-roles/doctors/training-doctor/foundation-training

NHS UK. Programmes [Internet]. UK Foundation Programme. Available from: https://foundationprogramme.nhs.uk/programmes/

Peninsula Deanery NHS UK. General Information on how Foundation training is organised - Peninsula Foundation [Internet]. Peninsuladeanery.nhs.uk. 2021 [cited 2024 Nov 12]. Available from: https://foundation.peninsuladeanery.nhs.uk/about-us/how-to-apply/two-year-programmes/recruitment-process/general-information-on-how-foundation-training-is-organised/

RCS England. Surgery Entry Requirements and Training [Internet]. Royal College of Surgeons. Available from: https://www.rcseng.ac.uk/careers-in-surgery/careers-support/what-is-surgery-like-as-a-career/entry-requirements-and-training/

4

The middle years: Core surgical training

INTRODUCTION

Core Surgical Training (CST) represents a pivotal moment in a trainee's surgical journey. It is the stage where you move beyond the foundations of medical training and begin to consciously shape yourself into a surgeon, developing not only technical proficiency, but also sound clinical judgement and the professional values that will underpin your future career in general surgery. The breadth of exposure to surgical subspecialties during CST provides you with a rich and formative grounding in the core principles of surgical practice.

As you move through this period, CST becomes a time of both challenge and growth. You will encounter steep learning curves, increasing responsibility, and moments that prompt reflection on your evolving professional identity. It is a stage that asks you to refine your skills, adapt to new ways of working, and learn from both successes and setbacks. Through this process, you begin to cultivate the confidence, resilience, and competence required to progress as a thoughtful and capable surgeon.

CORE SURGICAL TRAINEES WITHIN THE SENIOR HOUSE OFFICER FRAMEWORK

CST represent a structured evolution of the traditional senior house officer (SHO) role. Historically, SHOs occupied an intermediate grade between pre-registration house officers (PRHO) and Registrars, often with variable educational structure. This is demonstrated in Figure 3.1 in the previous chapter. Although the term "SHO" is now outdated within

DOI: 10.1201/9781003537663-4

formal training systems, it is still occasionally used informally to describe doctors working at this level.

Core surgical trainees can be viewed as a defined sub-group of this traditional SHO grade, distinguished by their placement on a nationally regulated surgical training pathway. While CSTs undertake many of the clinical and service responsibilities historically associated with SHOs, their roles are guided by a formal curriculum, clearly defined competencies, and structured assessment. As such, CST provides a more consistent and purposeful bridge between foundation training and higher surgical training.

APPLICATION FOR CORE SURGICAL TRAINING AND THE MULTI-SPECIALTY RECRUITMENT ASSESSMENT (MSRA)

CST is a structured, two-year postgraduate programme designed to provide resident doctors with broad-based experience across a range of surgical specialties, and in some instances, critical care. Following completion of the Foundation Programme, trainees enter CST through a competitive national selection process, which assesses clinical knowledge, aptitude, and commitment to a surgical career.

The application process for CST is coordinated nationally through the Oriel recruitment platform and involves several key components: completing the online application, sitting the MSRA, preparing a comprehensive surgical portfolio, and attending the selection interview.

The eligibility criteria, including essential and desirable requirements, are outlined on the NHS Careers and Health Education England (HEE) websites. As these criteria and the weighting of each selection component are reviewed annually, applicants are strongly encouraged to consult the most current guidance well in advance of the application cycle.

THE MULTI-SPECIALTY RECRUITMENT ASSESSMENT (MSRA)

The MSRA is a computer-based examination that forms an integral part of the national selection process for CST and several other postgraduate medical specialties. It comprises two sections:

1. *Professional Dilemmas (Situational Judgement Test)* – assessing professional integrity, empathy, and decision-making in realistic clinical scenarios.
2. *Clinical Problem Solving* – evaluating applied clinical knowledge across a broad range of specialties, reflecting the general medical foundation expected of all CST applicants.

The MSRA is offered at specific times each year, and successful completion within the application window is mandatory for consideration. Currently, MSRA scores are used for shortlisting candidates for interview and may also contribute to the final selection score, depending on national recruitment policy for that year.

Preparation and strategy

Effective preparation for the MSRA requires early planning and disciplined time management particularly when balancing revision alongside the demands of foundation training. A successful approach often includes the following:

- Early engagement with core material and revisiting fundamental clinical concepts
- Extensive question practice, using reputable MSRA-specific question banks to familiarise oneself with exam style, timing, and common themes
- Use of varied resources, such as clinical handbooks, revision courses, and peer study groups, to consolidate understanding and refine test-taking strategies
- Reflective learning, identifying weak areas early and targeting them through structured revision sessions

While preparation can be challenging, especially amidst clinical commitments, the MSRA is regarded as a fair and objective assessment. Candidates who maintain a broad, up-to-date clinical knowledge base and demonstrate sound professional judgement can confidently achieve competitive scores for CST shortlisting.

ROLES AND RESPONSIBILITIES OF CORE SURGICAL TRAINEES

During the two years of training, CSTs undertake rotations in various surgical subspecialties, such as general surgery, vascular surgery, orthopaedics, urology, ENT, and plastic surgery, as well as placements in intensive care or acute care settings. This diversity of experience equips trainees with the fundamental clinical, technical, and professional skills necessary for progression to higher surgical training in their chosen subspecialty.

CORE CLINICAL RESPONSIBILITIES

The role of CSTs is to provide essential day-to-day care for surgical inpatients and support the wider multidisciplinary team. The scope of responsibilities is broad and develops progressively with experience. Key duties include the following:

- *Inpatient and Ward Care*: Managing pre- and post-operative patients, conducting ward rounds, reviewing new admissions, and ensuring timely investigations and treatment plans. Core surgical trainees are expected to communicate effectively with patients and their families, maintain accurate documentation, and escalate concerns appropriately.
- *Emergency Surgical Take*: Participating in the acute surgical on-call rota, assessing new referrals, initiating appropriate management, and liaising with senior colleagues regarding urgent surgical decision-making. These shifts provide valuable exposure to undifferentiated surgical pathology and develop the trainee's clinical acumen and prioritisation skills.
- *Theatre and Procedural Experience*: Assisting and, where appropriate, performing basic surgical procedures under supervision in both elective and emergency operating lists. CSTs are encouraged to develop core operative competencies as outlined in the ISCP (Intercollegiate Surgical Curriculum Programme) and to actively seek supervised learning events to demonstrate progression.
- *Outpatient Clinics*: Participating in outpatient consultations to develop skills in clinical assessment, decision-making, and follow-up care. Clinics also provide opportunities to understand elective patient pathways from initial referral to surgical intervention.
- *Intensive Care and Perioperative Medicine (where applicable)*: In rotations involving intensive care or high-dependency units, trainees gain experience in managing critically ill patients, understanding perioperative optimisation, and developing procedural skills such as vascular access and airway management.

PROFESSIONAL DEVELOPMENT AND TEAM CONTRIBUTION

Beyond clinical duties, CSTs are expected to contribute to the broader functioning and development of their departments. This includes the following:

- Engaging in clinical audit, quality improvement, and research projects to enhance patient safety and service delivery

- Participating in teaching and supervision of medical students and junior colleagues
- Demonstrating commitment to leadership and management within the surgical environment
- Maintaining an up-to-date portfolio through the ISCP, documenting learning objectives, assessments, and reflections

THE CORE SURGICAL TRAINING (CST) CURRICULUM AND ASSESSMENTS

The CST curriculum provides a structured and outcomes-focused framework for resident doctors to develop the knowledge, clinical skills and professional behaviours expected of early stage surgical trainees. It is designed to give trainees a strong foundation in surgery before they move on to Higher Specialty Training (HST), which is more advanced training in a chosen surgical specialty.

The curriculum is managed by the Joint Committee for Surgical Training (JCST), which is the body responsible for overseeing surgical training in the UK. It is delivered through the ISCP, an online platform that guides learning, assessments, and progress tracking. The curriculum has been formally approved by the General Medical Council (GMC), the organisation that sets standards for doctors in the UK.

Trainees' progress over the two years of CST is recorded in the ISCP e-portfolio, which allows supervisors to give structured feedback, track assessments, and help trainees reflect on their learning and development.

Curriculum structure and frameworks

The CST curriculum is built around two key outcome frameworks:

- *Capabilities in Practice (CiPs)*: These are clinical tasks that describe what a surgeon needs to be able to do in everyday practice. There are five CiPs common to all surgical specialties:
  a. Managing outpatient clinics
  b. Managing the unselected emergency take
  c. Managing ward rounds and ongoing care of inpatients
  d. Managing an operating list
  e. Managing multidisciplinary team working

  Rather than assessing isolated skills through work-based assessments, CiPs reflect a broader judgement of overall performance. Each CiP integrates knowledge, clinical skills, technical skills, professional behaviours, and decision-making.

- *Generic Professional Capabilities (GPCs)*: These are the professional behaviours and values expected of all doctors, regardless of specialty. They include areas such as ethical practice, patient safety, communication skills, leadership, and teamwork.

Together, the CiPs and GPCs describe what trainees must be capable of doing at the end of their core training and provide a foundation for future progression.

Supervision levels

Progress in the curriculum is assessed not by counting individual tasks completed but by judging how much supervision a trainee needs to perform the CiPs safely. The CST curriculum defines several supervision levels, ranging from observation only (Level I) through to acting with direct supervision (Level II), and indirect supervision (Level III). As trainees develop, they are expected to require progressively less supervision in each CiP, which demonstrates increasing competence and readiness for more complex clinical responsibilities.

By the end of the two-year CST programme, trainees should normally be performing the CiPs at the expected supervision levels for core training Phase – for example, managing ward rounds and inpatient care under direct supervision and requiring less direct oversight for outpatient work and emergency take.

Supervision levels relating to consultant-level practice and beyond are deliberately excluded from the CST curriculum to ensure expectations remain appropriate for core trainees.

Workplace-based assessments (WBAs)

Formative WBAs are regular, low-stakes evaluations carried out during day-to-day clinical work. Their primary purpose is to support learning rather than to judge progression. They are based on direct observation and discussion, and they provide timely, constructive feedback to help trainees improve their skills and decision-making. By similarity to foundation training, a variety of WBAs may be undertaken, and these include the following:

- *Direct Observation of Procedural Skills (DOPS)*: assesses technical skills that can be observed in real time
- *Clinical Evaluation Exercises (CEXs)*: focuses on real-time clinical assessment and communication

- *Case-Based Discussions (CBDs)*: explores clinical reasoning and judgement in relation to a particular case
- *Procedure-Based Assessments (PBAs)*: assesses performance across entire surgical procedures
- *Multisource feedback*: gathers feedback on a trainee's performance and behaviours from various sources such as consultants, nurses, and other allied healthcare professionals

Together with the CiPs and GPCs, WBAs provide a comprehensive measure of the competencies outlined in the curriculum and support learning rather than determining progression.

Supervisors' reports

Trainees receive structured evaluations from consultants involved in their supervision, known as Multiple Consultant Reports (MCRs). These reports provide independent insights into performance across CiPs and GPCs, capturing progress in different clinical settings and under multiple supervisors. Each trainee also has an Assigned Educational Supervisor (AES) who monitors progress throughout the training year. The AES reviews all ISCP evidence, MCRs, and portfolio activity to produce a comprehensive report summarising strengths, development needs, and readiness to progress, alongside an overall narrative of the trainee's performance.

The annual review of competence progression (ARCP)

The ARCP is a formal review of evidence related to a trainee's progress throughout each stage of their specialty training. At the ARCP, a panel that includes the Training Programme Director uses the AES report, MCRs, and ISCP evidence to make a formal, high-stakes judgement on whether the trainee is ready to advance to the next stage. The panel considers overall capability, not just completion of individual tasks, ensuring that progression is based on consistent, well-rounded performance. The panel will decide on the outcome, such as Outcome 1 (achieving at the appropriate level) or a developmental outcome like Outcome 2, 3, or 4. For developmental outcomes, trainees are required to attend a feedback session to discuss the results and plan the next steps. If a trainee fails to provide existing documentation, they may receive an Outcome 5 and be required to attend a feedback panel to address the missing evidence. The ARCP would normally take place once a year for all trainees in surgical training. A panel may be convened more frequently for an interim review or to deal with progression issues.

MEMBERSHIP OF THE ROYAL COLLEGE OF SURGEONS (MRCS) AND PROGRESSION

Passing the MRCS examination, which comprises Part A (written) and Part B (clinical), is a key milestone during CST and a formal requirement for progression to higher surgical training (ST3). The MRCS assesses applied surgical knowledge, anatomy, pathology, and clinical acumen. Early preparation and consistent study alongside clinical duties are strongly advised (Figure 4.1).

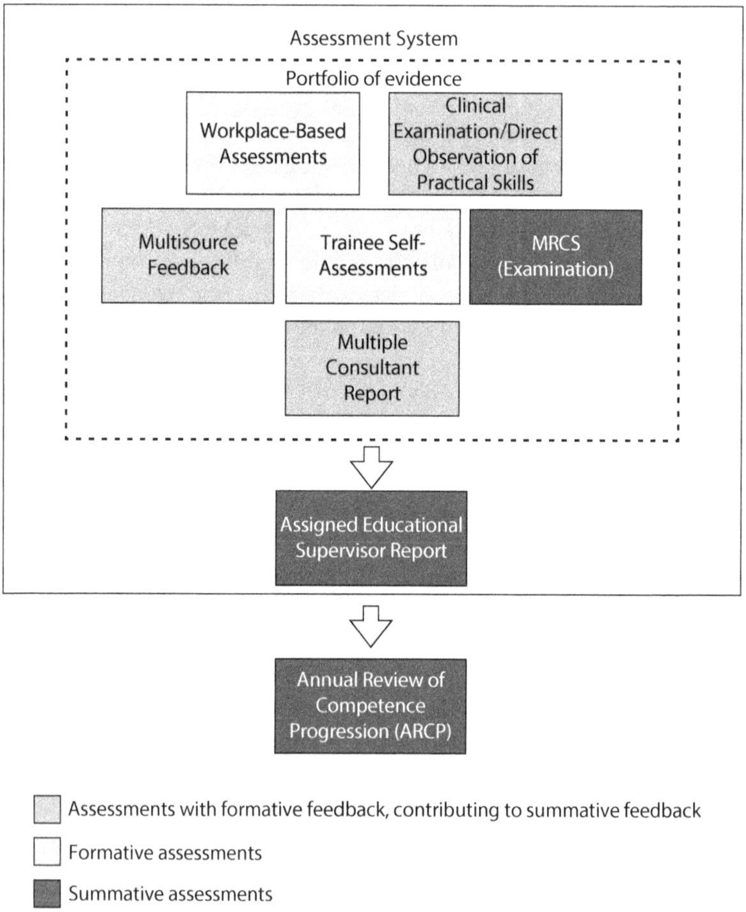

Figure 4.1 Assessment framework for CST.

CORE SURGICAL TRAINING SYLLABUS

Core surgical trainees are expected to demonstrate competence across a wide range of domains, including the following:

- *Basic Sciences*: A strong understanding of anatomy, physiology, pathology, microbiology, genetics, and related surgical sciences
- *Clinical Assessment and Decision-Making*: Competence in assessing, diagnosing, and formulating management plans for common surgical presentations; management of acutely unwell surgical patients; and contribution to the acute surgical take
- *Technical and Operative Skills*: Performing core surgical procedures such as wound closure and abscess drainage safely under supervision, and assisting effectively in more complex operations
- *Communication and Teamworking*: Building effective professional relationships with patients, colleagues, and the multidisciplinary team
- *Leadership and Management*: Taking initiative in clinical care, prioritising workloads, and contributing to team organisation
- *Professionalism and Ethics*: Upholding GMC standards of conduct, maintaining integrity, and demonstrating respect for patient dignity and autonomy
- *Teaching, Research, and Quality Improvement*: Engaging in teaching activities, audits, and quality improvement projects (QIPs) that enhance patient care and service efficiency

Training opportunities are delivered through a combination of elective operating lists, emergency on-call shifts, outpatient clinics, and ward-based learning. Each deanery or hospital may structure rotations differently, but all are required to provide adequate exposure to the core elements of the curriculum.

Where procedural opportunities are limited, trainees may be expected to utilise study leave, simulation training, or self-directed learning to complete required competencies. It is essential that trainees familiarise themselves with the most up-to-date ISCP curriculum corresponding to their year of entry, as requirements and expected competencies are periodically reviewed and updated.

Making the most of your general surgical placements

CST represents a demanding yet rewarding stage in your professional development. Balancing busy clinical rotas, on-call commitments, and study for postgraduate examinations can be challenging. However, with proactive engagement and thoughtful planning, your general surgical placements can provide invaluable learning opportunities that lay the foundation for a successful surgical career. To make the most of your general surgical placements.

BE PROACTIVE IN THE OPERATING THEATRE

The operating theatre is one of the most valuable learning environments in CST. While it is unrealistic to expect extensive operative exposure from the outset, enthusiasm, reliability, and attention to detail go a long way in earning the trust of senior colleagues.

- *Demonstrate Initiative*: Arrive prepared, know each patient's history, the indication for surgery, the anatomy and the key steps of the procedure.
- *Be a Conscientious Assistant*: Anticipate the needs of the operating team and maintain a high standard of asepsis and professionalism. This will improve with time and exposure.
- *Seek Opportunities Appropriately*: Not every operation lends itself to teaching. Recognise when efficiency and patient safety take precedence, but in suitable cases, discuss your learning goals beforehand such as inserting ports or closing wounds.
- *Reflect and Consolidate*: After each case, review the anatomy, techniques, and decision-making involved. Ask for feedback from your supervising surgeon to guide your progression.

Remember, CST is about developing a solid foundation. Building competence and confidence as a safe, reliable assistant is the first step towards becoming an effective operator.

EMBRACE THE FULL SPECTRUM OF SURGICAL LEARNING

Surgical training extends beyond the operating theatre. Equally important are the non-operative elements of patient care, which develop your clinical judgement and holistic understanding of surgery.

- *Ward and Inpatient Care*: Gain confidence in managing pre- and post-operative patients, in recognising complications early, and coordinating care with allied professionals.
- *Acute Surgical Take*: Use on-call shifts to refine your assessment skills, prioritise acutely unwell patients, and learn from decision-making in real time.
- *Critical Care and MDT Working*: Engage actively in multidisciplinary meetings and critical care rounds as these experiences strengthen your understanding of perioperative management and teamwork.

Exposure to these aspects of surgery will make you a more rounded and adaptable clinician, capable of seeing the bigger picture of surgical care.

FOSTER A COLLABORATIVE AND SUPPORTIVE APPROACH

CST can feel like a significant step-up in responsibility. However, it is vital to remember that you are part of a wider surgical team.

- *Seek Help Early*: Never hesitate to ask for guidance or clarification. Knowing your limitations is a mark of professionalism, not weakness.
- *Support Your Colleagues*: Collaborate with peers on audits, QIPs, and exam preparation. Shared learning fosters teamwork and helps build lasting professional relationships.
- *Maintain Professionalism*: Treat every team member: consultants, nurses, theatre staff, and juniors with respect and courtesy. Strong working relationships contribute to a positive learning environment and effective patient care.

CST is as much about developing your professional identity as it is about gaining technical skill. Collegiality, humility, and collaboration are qualities that will serve you throughout your surgical career.

APPROACH EACH PLACEMENT WITH PURPOSE

Each rotation offers a unique opportunity to develop specific skills and insights. Take time early in each placement to review the ISCP learning objectives, discuss your goals and learning agreements with your supervisor, and plan how to achieve them. Keep a reflective log of your progress, noting key cases, feedback, and lessons learned.

By engaging proactively, seeking feedback, and contributing positively to your team, you will not only maximise your learning but also establish yourself as a capable, dependable, and motivated trainee.

SUITABLE COURSES, CONFERENCES, AND PROFESSIONAL DEVELOPMENT

Attendance at structured courses and active participation in research, audits, and teaching are essential to demonstrate commitment to the specialty and prepare for higher surgical training. Core surgical trainees are required to attend regular regional teaching sessions organised by their deanery, which are provided free of charge and are mandatory. Attendance is essential for ARCP progression.

In addition to these compulsory sessions, there are several recommended courses and training opportunities specifically designed to support the development of competencies at the CST level.

KEY RECOMMENDED COURSES

- *Basic Surgical Skills (BSS)*: The Basic Surgical Skills course is a two-day introductory programme designed to teach safe surgical practice for late foundation and early core trainees. It covers essential open and minimally invasive techniques, including scrubbing, instrument handling, incision and drainage, biopsy, and basic laparoscopic procedures. Completion of BSS is often a prerequisite for progression to higher surgical training.
- *Advanced Trauma Life Support (ATLS)*: ATLS is an internationally recognised two-day course providing a structured, systematic approach to the management of trauma patients. Using the A–E framework, it combines pre-course study, simulation-based teaching, and practical assessments. Trainees gain experience in critical procedures such as chest drain insertion, surgical airways, and trauma resuscitation, making it a valuable credential for both on-call and emergency care settings.
- *Care of the Critically Ill Surgical Patient (CCrISP)*: Developed by the Royal College of Surgeons, CCrISP focuses on decision-making and the management of acutely unwell surgical patients. Delivered over two days, the course integrates case-based learning, data interpretation, and simulated patient scenarios to strengthen critical care reasoning and confidence in high-stakes environments.
- *Core Skills in Laparoscopic Surgery*: This practical course develops foundational competence in laparoscopic techniques through simulation and hands-on workshops, helping trainees build familiarity with key laparoscopic instruments and ergonomics.
- *Other Courses*: Additional courses, such as Advanced Paediatric Life Support (APLS) for paediatric-focused trainees, may be suitable alternatives or complements to the core surgical curriculum. Trainees are encouraged to attend courses aligned with their career goals and preparation for ST3 applications e.g. Trauma Basic Courses for aspiring orthopaedic surgeons and Duplex Ultrasound Training for aspiring vascular surgeons.

BUILDING A COMPETITIVE PORTFOLIO

- *Research and Academic Involvement*: Progression to higher surgical training is highly competitive. Developing a strong academic and research profile can significantly enhance your application. Trainees should aim to participate in ongoing research, submit work for presentation, and publish where possible. Presenting at national or regional conferences, whether as a poster, abstract, or oral presentation, demonstrates initiative and engagement with the surgical community. For those with academic aspirations, this experience can provide a foundation for future academic clinical fellowships or doctoral (PhD/MD) programmes.

- *Audits and QIPs*: Completing and closing the loop on at least one audit or QIP per year is strongly recommended. Projects can be identified through supervisors, departmental meetings, or personal observation of clinical practice. Starting early ensures time to analyse data, implement change, and demonstrate measurable improvement which is a key criterion for portfolio scoring and professional development.
- *Prizes, Grants, and Competitions*: Engagement with national surgical societies such as the Association of Surgeons in Training (ASiT), Royal Society of Medicine (RSM), and the Dukes' Club offers opportunities to apply for prizes, bursaries, and travel grants. Success in these areas not only enhances your portfolio but also provides valuable experience in research presentation and academic funding applications.

MAXIMISING LEARNING IN NON-GENERAL SURGICAL ROTATIONS

CSTs may rotate through a variety of non-general surgical specialties, such as trauma and orthopaedics, urology, otolaryngology (ENT), cardiothoracic surgery, plastic surgery, and intensive care medicine. These rotations complement general surgical training by providing valuable transferable skills and broadening clinical experience.

Even if a trainee's primary interest lies in general surgery, active engagement in these placements enhances both technical and non-technical abilities.

- *Urology*: Offers experience with endoscopic techniques and catheter management – skills applicable to the general surgeon
- *Intensive Care Medicine*: Builds competence in managing critically ill and post-operative patients, facilitates acquisition of transferable practical skills such as central line and chest drain insertion
- *ENT and Cardiothoracic Surgery*: Improves anatomical understanding, airway management, and precision in operative technique

Approaching each rotation with curiosity and initiative helps maximise learning and develop a well-rounded surgical skill set. The diverse exposure gained through CST cultivates clinical confidence and professionalism which are core attributes for success in higher surgical training.

PREPARING FOR ST3 APPLICATIONS

By the conclusion of CST, trainees are expected to have developed a broad and balanced surgical foundation, a comprehensive portfolio, and the professional maturity required to apply for ST3-level specialty training. This stage is critical for refining career goals, consolidating operative skills, and demonstrating the competence necessary for independent surgical decision-making.

CST also provides an ideal opportunity to strategically prepare for ST3 applications, which are highly competitive and assessed through portfolio review and interviews. Trainees should familiarise themselves with the current person specification for general surgery ST3 posts, available on the NHS and HEE websites. Similar to CST entry, ST3 applications typically require evidence of

- clinical and surgical experience;
- academic engagement, including research;
- audit and QIPs; and
- teaching and educational involvement.

Recommended preparatory resources include the guidebook *Cracking the General Surgical Interviews for ST3*, a title by the lead author of this book, and other structured interview preparation courses tailored to surgical specialties.

Successful completion of the MRCS examination is a mandatory prerequisite for progression to ST3. Although challenging, it is achievable with careful planning alongside full-time clinical commitments. The exam evaluates generalist surgical knowledge across multiple subspecialties.

MRCS Part A

- A written, multiple-choice examination assessing anatomy, physiology, pathology, and clinical knowledge.
- Can be attempted from FY1 onwards, though preparation requires significant time and consistent study.

MRCS Part B

- An OSCE-based assessment comprising 17–18 stations, including viva, surgical skills, history-taking, clinical examination, and critical care scenarios.
- Evaluates communication, clinical reasoning, procedural competence, and prioritisation skills in a practical, structured format.

Preparation resources include the following:

- RCS-approved courses and workshops
- Anatomy and surgical skills courses
- Online question banks and study materials

Early and consistent preparation for both MRCS and ST3 applications is essential. Combining portfolio development, audit and research activity, and operative skill consolidation positions trainees for a successful transition to HST.

CONCLUSION

CST is one of the most important stages in your surgical journey: a time when you move from learning the foundations of medicine to actively shaping yourself as a surgeon. During these two years, you will be exposed to a variety of surgical specialties and practical challenges that will test and expand both your technical skills and your clinical judgement. It is natural to feel both excitement and pressure at this stage; this is part of the process of growth. Approach every opportunity with curiosity and engagement. Be present in theatre, clinics, and ward rounds, but also take the time to reflect on what you see and do. Ask yourself not just "How do I perform this skill?" but also "Why am I making this decision?", and "How can I do better next time?" These moments of reflection are as important as hands-on experience. They are what transform technical competence into thoughtful, confident practice. Embrace teamwork. Learn from the consultants, senior trainees, nurses, and allied health professionals around you. Listen actively, communicate clearly, and support your colleagues; the relationships you build now will shape the professional environment you thrive in for years to come.

BIBLIOGRAPHY

Blacker T. Core surgery | health education England East Midlands [Internet]. Eastmidlandsdeanery.nhs.uk. 2018 [cited 2024 Nov 12]. Available from: https://www.eastmidlandsdeanery.nhs.uk/surgery/core_surgery

Brecknell J, Lintott P. Educating the surgeons of the future Curriculum Core Surgical Training THE INTERCOLLEGIATE SURGICAL CURRICULUM PROGRAMME Acknowledgements [Internet]. 2021 Aug. Available from: https://www.iscp.ac.uk/media/1111/core-surgical-training-curriculum-aug-2021-approved-oct-20.pdf

GMC UK. General surgery curriculum [Internet]. Gmc-uk.org. 2024. Available from: https://www.gmc-uk.org/education/standards-guidance-and-curricula/curricula/general-surgery-curriculum

Health Education England. Overview of Core Surgery Training CT1/ST1 | Workforce, training and education [Internet]. Workforce, training and education | Medical Hub. Available from: https://medical.hee.nhs.uk/medical-training-recruitment/medical-specialty-training/surgery/core-surgery/overview-of-core-surgery-training/overview-of-core-training

Health Education Northwest. Global Objectives and ARCP Requirements for North West Core Surgical resident doctors | Health Education North West [Internet]. Nwpgmd.nhs.uk. 2021 [cited 2024 Nov 12]. Available from: https://www.nwpgmd.nhs.uk/Specialty_Schools/Surgery/Core_Surgical_Training/ARCP_Requirements

JCST. Core surgical training [Internet]. JCST. Available from: https://www.jcst.org/uk-trainees/core-surgical-training/

RCS England. Basic surgical skills (Intercollegiate BSS) [Internet]. Royal College of Surgeons. Available from: https://www.rcseng.ac.uk/education-and-exams/courses/search/basic-surgical-skills-intercollegiate-bss/

RCS England. Surgery Entry Requirements and Training [Internet]. Royal College of Surgeons. Available from: https://www.rcseng.ac.uk/careers-in-surgery/careers-support/what-is-surgery-like-as-a-career/entry-requirements-and-training/

RCS Ireland. Core surgical training – Overview [Internet]. www.rcsi.com. Available from: https://www.rcsi.com/surgery/training/surgery/cst/overview

5

The later years: Higher surgical training

INTRODUCTION

Higher Specialty Training (HST) represents the advanced phase of surgical education that follows completion of Core Surgical Training (CST). As the final and most extensive stage of postgraduate surgical training, HST is often described as a period of consolidation and increasing responsibility, gradually shaping doctors into confident, independent consultants within their chosen surgical specialty.

Trainees may pursue one of ten recognised surgical subspecialties: General Surgery, Cardiothoracic Surgery, Neurosurgery, Oral and Maxillofacial Surgery, Otolaryngology, Paediatric Surgery, Plastic Surgery, Trauma and Orthopaedics, Urology, and Vascular Surgery. With the exception of Neurosurgery, which follows a run-through training pathway beginning at Specialty Training level 1 (ST1), most surgical specialties recruit trainees upon successful completion of the CST programme. Doctors who commenced HST in the UK on or after 1 August 2007 are designated as Specialty Registrars (StRs). This chapter will specifically focus on HST in General Surgery.

RECRUITMENT INTO HIGHER SPECIALTY TRAINING (HST) IN GENERAL SURGERY

Entry into HST in General Surgery is achieved through a nationally competitive selection process. This involves completing a formal application, compiling a comprehensive portfolio of surgical experience, and performing successfully at a structured interview.

DOI: 10.1201/9781003537663-5

The application form is designed to evaluate a candidate's suitability for entry into HST. To be longlisted, applicants must meet the minimum eligibility criteria outlined in the national person specification, which include the following:

- A recognised medical qualification (MBBS or equivalent)
- Completion of Parts A and B of the Membership Examination of the Royal College of Surgeons (MRCS) by the offer date
- A complete employment history
- Achievement of CST competencies or equivalent experience

Candidates are scored based on their surgical portfolio, which may include the following:

- Duration of experience in general and other surgical specialties
- Operative logbook (e.g. core procedures such as appendicectomies)
- Publications, presentations, audits, and quality improvement projects
- Higher degrees or additional qualifications

Notably, excessive time spent in General Surgery is penalised, as it may confer an unfair advantage over candidates who progressed through the CST pathway. The total score from the application determines shortlisting for the interview.

THE INTERVIEW PROCESS

The interview for entrance into HST, referred to commonly as the ST3 interview, is highly competitive. Candidates must achieve the best possible score to secure a National Training Number (NTN) and obtain their preferred post.

The interview format has evolved considerably over recent years. Prior to 2020, it comprised five stations assessing elements of the portfolio, clinical acumen, management scenarios, communication, and technical skills.

During the 2020 COVID-19 global pandemic, the process was suspended and replaced with portfolio self-assessment, with top-ranked candidates allocated posts based on verified scores.

From 2021 onwards, the self-assessment system was discontinued, and a streamlined structured interview was introduced. The current 40-minute interview consists of three stations, each aligned with the ST3 General Surgery person specification:

1. Clinical Station – 15 minutes
   The Clinical Station assesses a candidate's core clinical knowledge and their ability to apply this knowledge to common general surgical presentations. Candidates are usually presented with a short, focused scenario reflecting situations encountered on the acute surgical take, on the wards, or in outpatient clinics. The emphasis is on safe, structured clinical reasoning, including assessment, formulation of differential diagnoses, initial investigations, and immediate management. This station evaluates a candidate's grasp of fundamental surgical principles and ability to communicate their thought process clearly under time pressure.
2. Clinical Management Station – 15 minutes
   The Clinical Management Station differs from the Clinical Station in that it focuses on decision-making in a more complex scenario that involves a management dilemma. Candidates are expected to demonstrate an understanding of the wider clinical context, including multidisciplinary working, escalation of concerns, and effective use of available resources. Scenarios may explore issues such as balancing competing priorities, managing risk, addressing patient safety concerns, or responding to service pressures. This station assesses leadership potential, professionalism, situational awareness, and the ability to make pragmatic decisions while working within the realities of the healthcare system.
3. Portfolio Station – 10 minutes
   The Portfolio Station evaluates the quality of a candidate's portfolio, with particular focus on engagement in clinical governance and professional development. Candidates may be questioned on their involvement in audits, quality improvement projects, research, teaching, and leadership activities, as well as their understanding of key concepts such as audit cycles, research methodology, and governance principles. In addition, candidates may be asked to reflect on their strengths and areas for development. This station assesses commitment to ongoing improvement, insight into one's own practice, and readiness to contribute to the broader responsibilities of a higher surgical trainee.

Together, these three stations provide a balanced assessment of clinical competence, professional judgement, and evidence of career development. The interviews are now conducted on a standardised online platform, following the widespread adoption of telemedicine.

Key to success in securing a NTN

Success in this highly competitive interview process depends on a clear and detailed understanding of the person specification, coupled with thorough and purposeful preparation. Candidates who take the time to align their experience and achievements to the criteria in the person specification will be better equipped to present themselves convincingly and coherently at interview. This process is not simply about demonstrating competence but also about evidencing suitability for the next stage of training.

Preparation should begin early and be approached in a structured and methodical manner. A recruitment timeline, including the anticipated interview window, is usually published in the final quarter of the year preceding the recruitment cycle. This provides candidates with the opportunity to develop a focused preparation strategy over time. In addition to personal preparation, there are established resources designed specifically to support candidates through this process. These include dedicated interview preparation textbooks, notably *Cracking the General Surgical Interviews for ST3*, published in 2022, which provides structured guidance aligned to the interview format and expectations.

Given the structured nature of these interviews, deliberate and repeated practice is essential. Engaging in mock interviews with peers, senior colleagues, or mentors allows candidates to refine their responses, improve clarity, and gain constructive feedback. Formal interview preparation courses are also available and can offer targeted practice, exposure to realistic interview scenarios, and expert insight into common pitfalls and marking criteria. Such opportunities help candidates develop concise, well-structured answers that reflect both sound clinical knowledge and professional judgement.

Ultimately, candidates who are most successful at these interviews are those who prepare well, making effective use of preparation resources, and demonstrate at interview not only clinical knowledge but also reflective insight into their practice and future development.

TRAINING AND PROGRESSION DURING HIGHER SPECIALTY TRAINING (HST)

Higher Surgical Training in General Surgery is organised according to national standards that are designed to ensure a consistently high standard of training and professional development for surgeons across the UK. These standards set out what trainees are expected to learn, the skills they must develop, and the level of performance they must achieve before they can progress or complete training.

The detailed training plans, known as curricula and syllabuses, are written and regularly updated by a group of experienced surgeons called the Surgical Advisory Committee (SAC). These committees work in line with the General Medical Council (GMC), which is the national body responsible for setting the standards for doctors' training, competence, and professional behaviour. In simple terms, the GMC defines what a safe and effective doctor should be able to do, and the SAC ensures that surgical training meets these expectations.

There are ten different surgical specialties in the UK, such as General Surgery, Orthopaedics, and Neurosurgery, and each specialty has its own SAC. These specialty-specific committees are coordinated by a larger organisation called the Joint Committee on Surgical Training (JCST). The JCST brings together the four Surgical Royal Colleges of the UK and Ireland and acts as the central body that oversees and advises on all aspects of surgical training, helping to ensure that training is consistent, fair, and of high quality nationwide.

The training portfolio and assessment framework

The following section revisits topics that were discussed in detail in the CST chapter. Like CSTs, Specialty Registrars (StRs) in surgery are required to maintain an electronic training portfolio using the Intercollegiate Surgical Curriculum Programme (ISCP) platform. Introduced in 2007, the ISCP provides a single, structured system that brings together all aspects of surgical training. In practical terms, it acts as a central record of a trainee's progress, incorporating the approved curriculum in one section, the surgical logbook in another section, and a dedicated section for evidence from assessments completed throughout training.

As discussed in the chapter on CST, the key function of the ISCP is to support assessment and feedback. These assessments fall into two main categories: *formative* and *summative*.

Formative assessments are regular, low-stakes assessments carried out during day-to-day clinical work. Their primary purpose is to support learning rather than to judge progression. They are based on direct observation and discussion, and they provide timely, constructive feedback to help trainees improve their skills and decision-making. These work-based assessments (WBAs) include the following:

- *Direct Observation of Procedural Skills (DOPS)*: assesses technical skills that can be observed in real time
- *Clinical Evaluation Exercises (CEXs)*: focuses on real time clinical assessment and communication

- *Case-Based Discussions (CBDs)*: explores clinical reasoning and judgement in relation to a particular case
- *Procedure-Based Assessments (PBAs)*: assesses performance across entire surgical procedures
- *Multisource Feedback*: gathers feedback on a trainee's performance and behaviours from various sources such as consultants, nurses and other allied healthcare professionals

In contrast, summative assessments are high-stakes reviews that determine whether a trainee is ready to progress. The most important of these is the Annual Review of Competence Progression (ARCP). This is a formal, yearly process in which a panel reviews the trainee's portfolio evidence within the ISCP to assess progress against the curriculum requirements. The outcome of the ARCP determines whether the trainee can move on to the next stage of training, requires additional support, or needs further time to meet the expected standards.

Alongside these assessment processes, surgical training has been shaped by significant curriculum reform. In 2021, a new General Surgery curriculum was introduced, representing a move away from a purely "competency-based" mode toward an "outcome-based" approach. Under this system, the focus is not just on completing individual tasks or assessments, but on demonstrating the ability to perform key areas of professional practice safely and independently. The GMC defines an outcome as an area of practice that a trainee can be trusted to carry out without direct supervision.

Central to the new curriculum are *Capabilities in Practice* (CiPs). These describe the essential areas of work that a newly appointed consultant surgeon should be able to manage from their first day in post. Rather than assessing isolated skills through WBAs, CiPs reflect a broader judgement of overall performance, bringing together technical ability, clinical reasoning, communication, and professionalism. In General Surgery, the CiPs are grouped into four core domains:

1. Managing the unselected emergency surgical take
2. Running outpatient clinics
3. Managing ward rounds and inpatient care
4. Delivering safe operative care and managing patients before and after surgery
5. Working effectively within a multidisciplinary team

In addition to CiPs, trainees must demonstrate Generic Professional Capabilities (GPCs). These are the professional behaviours and values expected of all doctors, regardless of specialty. They include areas such as ethical practice, patient safety, communication skills, leadership, and teamwork.

Progression through HST is now based on demonstrated capability rather than simply time spent in post. While there are indicative timeframes for training, trainees who consistently show the required capabilities and professional behaviours may progress more quickly. This approach aims to produce surgeons who are not only technically competent, but also well-rounded and ready for independent practice.

Consultants who are involved directly in the supervision of a trainee will provide structured evaluations known as Multiple Consultant Reports (MCRs). Multiple Consultant Reports offer independent consultant perspectives on the trainee's performance across CiPs and GPCs. They provide important evidence of performance across different settings and supervisors.

Each trainee has an Assigned Educational Supervisor (AES) that oversees the trainee's progress over the training year, reviewing all ISCP evidence, MCRs, and portfolio activity. The AES uses this information to produce a comprehensive report that highlights strengths, areas for development, and readiness to progress, as well as a narrative of the trainee's overall performance.

The ARCP is a formal review of evidence related to a trainee's progress throughout each stage of their specialty training. At the ARCP, a panel that includes the Training Programme Director uses the AES report, MCRs, and ISCP evidence to make a formal, high-stakes judgement on whether the trainee is ready to advance to the next stage. The panel considers overall capability, not just completion of individual tasks, ensuring that progression is based on consistent, well-rounded performance. The ARCP would normally take place once a year for all trainees in surgical training. A panel may be convened more frequently for an interim review or to deal with progression issues.

In summary, CiPs and GPCs provide the framework for what a trainee must be able to do, while MCRs, AES reports, and the ISCP portfolio together supply the evidence that these capabilities are being achieved. The ARCP then formally integrates this evidence to confirm readiness for progression (Figure 5.1).

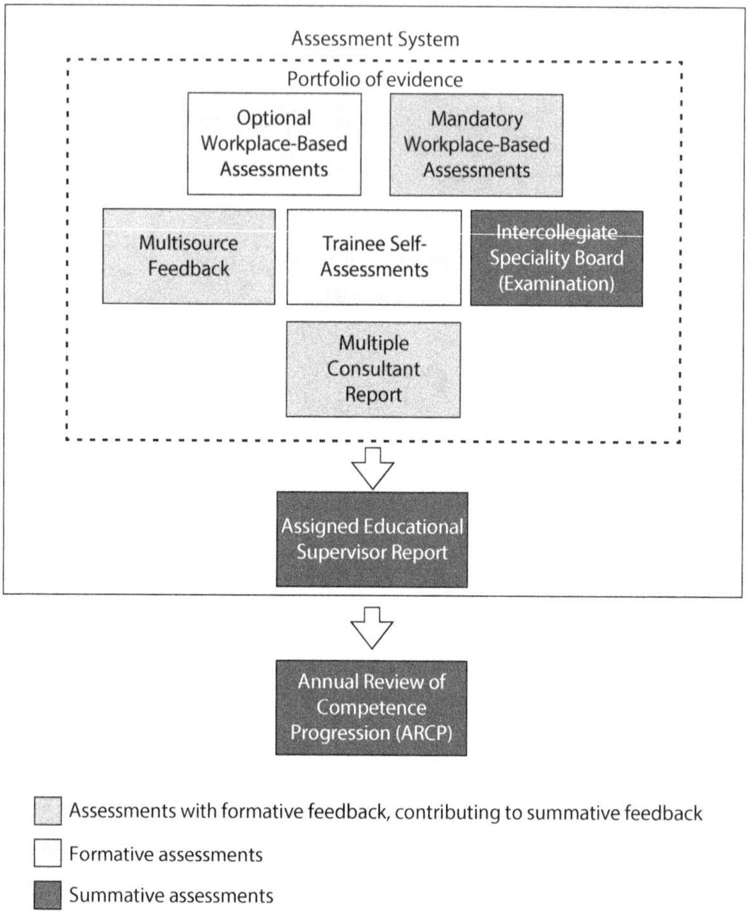

Figure 5.1 Assessment framework for HST.

The full general surgical curriculum is available on the ISCP website at www.iscp.ac.uk.

Completion of training

Upon successful completion of all training requirements and demonstration of the necessary capabilities, the trainee is awarded an Outcome 6 at their ARCP – signifying Completion of Training (CCT). The award of a CCT confers eligibility for entry onto the Specialist Register, enabling the surgeon to practise independently as a consultant.

MAXIMISING TRAINING OPPORTUNITIES DURING HIGHER SPECIALTY TRAINING (HST)

StRs in HST progress at varying rates, influenced by factors such as individual aptitude, prior experience, exposure, and the quality of their learning environment. The General Surgery curriculum provides an outline of the expected pace of capability acquisition. StRs are strongly encouraged to familiarise themselves with this curriculum and to remain actively engaged with ISCP throughout their training journey.

Progress and success in HST depend equally on the initiative of the trainee and the supportiveness of the training environment. While service commitments within the NHS can sometimes overshadow training opportunities, clinical service and learning are not mutually exclusive. With proactive planning, time management, and engagement, trainees can balance their duties to patients with consistent professional development.

Creating a Personal Development Plan (PDP) at the beginning of each rotation is very important. It helps trainees clearly set out what they want to learn and plan the steps needed to achieve these goals. The PDP acts like a roadmap for learning, showing what knowledge and skills need to be developed during the rotation. Reviewing and updating the plan from time to time is essential, as this keeps the learning on track.

The following sections outline practical strategies for maximising learning and skill development in each core area of the 2021 General Surgery curriculum.

Outpatient clinics

- Undertake triage of GP referrals under supervision to enhance decision-making and prioritisation skills.
- Discuss clinic cases and management plans with supervising consultants to demonstrate clinical reasoning, diagnostic acumen, and communication skills.
- Request consultant review of clinic letters to refine documentation and case summarisation.
- Aim to complete WBAs for as many patient encounters as feasible.

Ward work and inpatient care

- Ask your supervising consultant to observe your ward rounds and provide feedback on:
  - patient prioritisation and escalation;
  - leadership and delegation within the multidisciplinary team;
  - clinical assessment, interpretation of results, and discharge planning;

  - documentation quality; and
  - situational awareness
- Engage in regular WBAs to consolidate these skills

The unselected emergency take

- Request consultant observation and feedback on your ability to:
  - rapidly assess and stabilise acutely unwell patients;
  - prioritise cases according to clinical urgency;
  - apply protocols such as ATLS;
  - manage comorbidities in acute surgical presentations;
  - select and initiate appropriate conservative or operative management;
  - coordinate with anaesthetists, intensivists, and other MDT members;
  - conduct post-operative care and ensure accurate documentation; and
  - use on-call shifts as rich opportunities for WBAs and targeted feedback.

The operating list

- Discuss patient selection and list preparation with consultants; where possible, arrange for procedures requiring more experience to be included in your lists.
- Review clinic notes and imaging before operating lists to demonstrate preparedness and initiative.
- Prioritise continuity of supervision, as repeated guidance from the same consultant enhances technical and cognitive learning.
- Use downtime to revise anatomy and discuss procedural steps to reinforce understanding.
- Request observation and feedback on pre-operative briefings, application of the WHO surgical checklist, and intraoperative performance.
- Work collaboratively with co-registrars to share learning opportunities.
- Engage in theatre efficiency: assist in preparing the next case and streamline workflow to maximise operative exposure.
- Write operation notes for cases you assisted or performed – this reinforces learning and documentation skills.
- Consider private assisting opportunities to expand procedural familiarity.
- Observe other surgeons to develop insight into technique and operative style.
- Value all cases, including minor operations, as opportunities to refine skills.

Multidisciplinary team (MDT) working

- Take ownership of selected cases and lead MDT discussions when appropriate.
- Seek consultant feedback on presentation skills, collaboration, and management of differing opinions.
- Ensure accurate documentation and arrangement of follow-up plans.

Training and education

- Engage in simulation and skills practice: utilise laparoscopic trainers, hospital skills labs, and practice basic techniques such as knot tying.
- Attend Royal College of Surgeons-accredited courses, such as the following:
  - Intermediate Skills in Laparoscopic Surgery
  - ATLS Reverification and Instructor Courses
  - Care of the Critically Ill Surgical Patient (CCrISP) Instructor Course
  - Clinical Skills in Emergency Surgery
  - Training the Trainers
- Prepare for the FRCS through established courses (e.g. Whipps Cross, Alpine).
- Join relevant specialty associations (ACPGBI, AUGIS, BOMMS, British Hernia Society, ASiT, WINS) to access resources, courses, and research opportunities.
- Consider pursuing higher degrees (MD, PhD, MBA) or fellowships (research, global surgery) to broaden experience.
- Maintain an updated portfolio of audits, QI projects, and research.

Leadership and management

- Undertake formal leadership and management courses or participate in activities that foster these skills, such as the following:
  - Organising teaching programmes or trainee forums
  - Acting as a regional trainee representative
  - Managing rotas or operating lists
  - Exploring structured opportunities such as the RCS Emerging Leaders Programme

Professionalism

- Revisit the GMC's Good Medical Practice guidance and updates regularly.
- Attend courses on teamwork, ethics, and communication offered by the GMC or indemnity providers.
- Participate in human factors training to enhance safety and situational awareness.

Meetings with supervisors

- Supervision is central to training. Build productive relationships with your clinical and educational supervisors.
- Prepare in advance for meetings to ensure focused discussions and effective feedback.
- Schedule regular meetings throughout the rotation rather than clustering them near the end.
- Raise challenges early and collaboratively seek solutions.

Planning rotations and the ARCP

- Take an active role in managing your training – your initiative drives your progress. The Training Programme Director (TPD) supports and directs your development.
- Map out desired experiences and plan rotations strategically.
- Be adaptable in relocation for training opportunities; balance professional growth with personal considerations.
- Identify mentors who value teaching and aim to spend time in their units.
- Keep your ISCP portfolio up to date, ensuring all sign-offs and documentation are completed before the ARCP.

Additional considerations

- Financial Support: Health Education England provides a relocation budget of up to £8,000, which can offset costs associated with training moves – a resource not widely advertised but highly beneficial.
- Philanthropy and Global Surgery: Engage in charitable surgical work (e.g. Operation Hernia, Operation International UK, Médecins Sans Frontières). These experiences foster global awareness and broaden clinical perspective and experience.

FINAL THOUGHTS

Excellence in surgical training is achieved through a blend of personal initiative, reflective practice, and purposeful engagement with every learning opportunity. Only by remaining proactive and adaptable can surgical trainees maximise the value of their HST years, developing not only as competent surgeons but also as future leaders in healthcare.

To make the most of your HST journey:

- *Be proactive*: Seek out every opportunity to learn, both inside and outside the operating theatre. Take initiative in your own development and actively engage with your training programme.
- *Start early*: Build a strong foundation of surgical knowledge and technical skills as soon as possible. Stay current with evolving clinical guidelines and best practices.
- *Be present*: Surgery is a hands-on discipline best learned through experience and observation. Even when not scrubbed in, there is much to gain from closely watching senior colleagues and understanding their decision-making processes.
- *Engage in continuous learning*: Attend courses, pursue additional skills, and apply new techniques thoughtfully in clinical practice.
- *Develop your portfolio*: Familiarise yourself with your curriculum, maintain an accurate and detailed logbook, and regularly update your ISCP portfolio with evidence of clinical activity, reflection, and achievement.

Ultimately, your surgical training is what you make of it. The direction and depth of your experience depend largely on your initiative and engagement. Take ownership of your journey, cultivate curiosity, seek feedback, and embrace every challenge. In doing so, you will not only refine your surgical expertise but also shape yourself into a well-rounded, reflective, and resilient clinician.

BIBLIOGRAPHY

Gold guide 10th Edition: Postgraduate foundation and specialty training in the UK. Version: GG10 7th August 2024.

General Surgery – Higher Surgical Training (ST3), NHS England / Health Education England Medical. https://medical.hee.nhs.uk/medical-training-recruitment/medical-specialty-training/surgery/higher-surgery/general-surgery/overview-of-general-surgery/overview-of-general-surgery?utm_source=copilot.com

Intercollegiate Surgical Curriculum Programme (ISCP). General Surgery Curriculum. Version 2, August 2021 (updated July 2023).

6

Preparing for consultant practice

INTRODUCTION

For many aspiring surgeons, becoming a consultant feels like the culmination of years of effort, sacrifice, and determination, much like reaching the summit of a mountain after a long and demanding climb. The journey requires careful preparation, resilience in the face of setbacks, and the stamina to keep going when the path feels steep and uncertain. Those who reach this stage do so having been shaped by the challenges along the way, emerging not only as skilled clinicians but also as leaders within the healthcare system, entrusted with delivering and shaping patient care.

Unlike a mountain climb, however, there is no descent after reaching this peak. Stepping into a consultant role represents a profound and lasting transition. It is a moment of growth and reinvention, where responsibility deepens, specialist interests take clearer shape, and professional identity truly settles. The rewards, both personal and professional, are significant, reflecting the years of commitment, perseverance, and passion that have brought surgeons to this point.

DEVELOPING SKILLS TO THE LEVEL OF A DAY-1 CONSULTANT

The journey to becoming a consultant surgeon in the UK is a structured and rigorous process, outlined in detail in previous chapters. In summary, after graduating from medical school, aspiring surgeons undertake two years of Foundation Training, gaining broad clinical experience across multiple medical specialties. This is followed by Core Surgical Training

DOI: 10.1201/9781003537663-6

(CST), where the focus narrows to surgical disciplines, establishing a solid foundation in the fundamental principles and skills of surgery.

The most critical phase is Higher Surgical Training (HST), during which trainees immerse themselves deeply into their chosen surgical specialty. This stage is designed to equip aspiring surgeons with the advanced knowledge, technical expertise, and professional judgement necessary to function confidently at the level of a day-1 consultant. Successful completion of this phase of training culminates in the award of the Certificate of Completion of Training (CCT), a distinguished credential that formally recognises consultant-level competence and grants entry onto the specialist register.

In preparation for independent practice, trainees may be authorised to "act up" as consultants during the final three months prior to the award of CCT, subject to approval by their training deanery. This period allows a trainee to begin inhabiting the role of a consultant while still benefiting from an element of supervision and support. Acting up allows trainees to experience the realities of consultant practice firsthand: leading clinical decision-making, managing increased responsibility, and navigating the broader professional expectations that extend beyond technical expertise. It also offers a valuable opportunity to test one's readiness and build confidence in a real-world setting.

This transitional phase enables surgeons to step into their future role gradually, consolidating their identity as independent practitioners while still having the reassurance of oversight. For many, it becomes a formative experience, one that not only eases the transition but also shapes how they will practise as consultants in the years to come.

POST-CCT FELLOWSHIPS

A post-CCT fellowship is a period of additional, specialised training that a surgeon can do after completing their official surgical training (CCT). Think of it as an extra year or two to focus on a specific area of surgery, like colorectal, upper GI, or hernia surgery, and gain experience with more complex cases. During a fellowship, the surgeon works in a hospital or centre of excellence, sometimes abroad, under the guidance of experienced consultants where exposure to complex pathology, high-volume practice, and advanced techniques is both concentrated and immersive. For many surgeons, post-CCT fellowships offer a meaningful pause before full consultant practice, a period of deliberate refinement of knowledge and skills in a chosen subspecialty. Having completed the core requirements of training, these fellowships provide the space to deepen expertise beyond the standard curriculum and to pursue areas of genuine passion with focus and intent.

The competitive nature of post-CCT fellowships reflects their important value. Funding and support for post-CCT fellowships are often available through NHS England, regional health education bodies, and professional surgical colleges, helping to make these opportunities accessible. Whether undertaken in the UK or abroad, post-CCT fellowships represent a significant investment in professional growth, one that allows surgeons to emerge more confident and specialised.

SEARCHING FOR CONSULTANT POSTS

As trainees approach the completion of their CCT or post-CCT fellowship, proactive planning for securing a consultant position is essential. The primary platform for consultant recruitment in England and Wales is the NHS Jobs website, which advertises vacancies across NHS trusts. Many organisations also post opportunities on their own websites. Additionally, consultant posts may be found through national publications such as the *BMJ*, recruitment agencies, job search engines like Indeed.com, and professional networking platforms, including LinkedIn. Trainees may also find out about consultant posts through word of mouth. What's important is that early and strategic job searching, combined with networking, can significantly enhance the prospects of securing a suitable consultant appointment.

PREPARING FOR CONSULTANT INTERVIEWS

Often seen as one of the most important and challenging interviews in a surgeon's career, the consultant interview marks a key turning point. It is a chance to reflect on your journey, showcase your skills and experience, and demonstrate your readiness to take on a leadership role in healthcare. Preparing thoughtfully and dedicating time and effort to this process can make a real difference. The following guidance is offered to support aspiring consultants as they approach this important stage.

Mastering the application process

- *Timing and Application Completion*: Consultant applications are typically submitted online via the NHS Jobs portal. Allocate sufficient time to complete your application thoroughly and thoughtfully because rushed submissions risk omission or error. Late applications are not accepted. Ensure your Curriculum Vitae (CV) is current and meticulously tailored to the specific post, emphasising relevant experience and competencies.

- *Job Description and Person Specification*: Review these very carefully to understand the clinical responsibilities, desired attributes, and expectations for the role. Your personal statement should clearly articulate why you are the ideal candidate and what unique contributions you can bring to the unit or trust. Conduct thorough background research on the trust and department, as this insight will inform a compelling, targeted application.

Pre-interview preparation and site visit

- *Understanding the Trust and Department*: Upon invitation to interview, deepen your research on the trust's values, clinical services and strategic priorities. Even if familiar with the organisation, reviewing the latest trust Annual Report and Care Quality Commission (CQC) assessments, usually available on the trust website, will provide valuable context and demonstrate your engagement with broader organisational goals.
- *Interview Panel Insight*: Information about panel members is often provided with interview invitations. Typical panels for permanent consultant posts include clinical leaders (Clinical or Divisional Directors), trust executives, human resources representatives, and Royal College of Surgeons representatives. Arrange a pre-interview visit to meet panel members if possible. Use this opportunity to glean insights into the department's culture and challenges and to subtly showcase your credentials. Prepare thoughtful questions about the trust's future strategy and the specialty's role, which can be woven into your interview responses to highlight your preparedness and genuine interest.

Interview day strategy

- *Professional Presentation*: Dress appropriately, even for virtual interviews, and approach the day with calm confidence. You may be asked to deliver a presentation, so prepare carefully to communicate your vision and value effectively.
- *Typical Questions*: Initial questions are often straightforward: examples include why you want the role, what you bring to the position, and how you stand out from other candidates. Prepare to address clinical scenarios and risk management issues, reflecting your depth of knowledge and judgement.
- *Behavioural Examples*: Have concrete examples ready to demonstrate your leadership, teamwork, communication skills, problem-solving abilities, and self-awareness regarding your strengths and areas for development.

THE REALITY OF CONSULTANT LIFE

Congratulations, you've secured the post! This marks a significant career achievement, but it also ushers in new responsibilities and challenges. Understanding both the rewards and realities will help you navigate this transition successfully.

- *The highlights*:
  - Enjoy a more predictable and stable schedule, with greater control over your working pattern compared to training rotations.
  - Greater autonomy enables you to balance clinical work with personal priorities and explore roles in education, leadership, research, and outreach.
- *New territories*:
  - The shift to independent practice carries ultimate responsibility for patient care, which can be daunting initially. Seek support and second opinions from trusted colleagues. Consultancy does not mean isolation.
  - Administrative duties and bureaucracy are inevitable. Ensure your job plan allocates at least 1.5 SPA (Supporting Professional Activities) sessions weekly to manage these effectively.
  - The annual appraisal is a tool for continuous professional development. Requires time and effort. Start early and document evidence throughout the year.
  - Industry representatives may approach you with product promotions – maintain a professional but discerning approach, prioritising evidence-based practice.
- *Day-to-day working environment*:
  - Your success relies on strong relationships with your multidisciplinary team: colleagues, resident doctors, nurses, administrative staff, theatre teams, and allied health professionals. Cultivate respect, humility, and open communication.
  - Workplace dynamics vary; be prepared to navigate and diffuse conflicts with empathy and a patient-centred focus.
  - Recognise and appreciate the contributions of all team members, including support staff, who play vital roles in delivering patient care.
  - Be prepared to address any discrimination or bias, including those related to gender, race, disability, or intersectional factors. Know your rights and the support systems available.
- *Well-being and resilience*:
  - The privilege of caring for patients is balanced by significant pressures. Prioritise your mental health by maintaining a healthy work-life balance and nurturing relationships outside work.

LOCUM CONSULTANT POSTS

Locum consultant posts are increasingly common within the NHS and are often viewed as a valuable pathway toward securing a permanent consultant position. These roles are advertised similarly to permanent posts, though the interview process tends to be less formal and involves a smaller panel. Locum positions are typically offered for six months to one year and may serve a variety of purposes: providing cover for a consultant on extended leave or sabbatical or acting as a stepping stone toward a permanent appointment.

For trainees, locum roles offer a unique opportunity to practice at a consultant level while retaining the flexibility to move on if desired. For trusts and departments, these positions can function as an extended trial period, allowing both parties to assess suitability before committing to a permanent appointment. Overall, locum consultancy offers a mutually beneficial arrangement, blending professional development with operational flexibility.

SUMMARY

A career as a consultant offers immense rewards, providing the opportunity to shape your professional journey in alignment with your passions and ambitions. While many of the challenges experienced during training may lessen, you will inevitably encounter a new set of demands, each presenting an opportunity for growth and personal development.

Do not hesitate to seek guidance when needed, and value the trusted colleagues and mentors who can offer perspective and support. Foster a collaborative spirit, prioritise the well-being of your team, and cultivate a positive, inclusive workplace culture. Such an approach not only enhances team performance but also enables those around you to reach their full potential. Recognise that certain aspects of your journey will be personal and some goals are deeply individual. Prioritising your mental health is essential, as sustained well-being underpins long-term professional success. Live according to your values and lead by example, as this is the hallmark of exemplary surgical leadership.

BIBLIOGRAPHY

ID medical – . The Journey to Becoming an NHS Consultant. Published 5 February 2024.

Ross J. Preparing for your first consultant job. The Medical Defence Union (MDU). Published 18 July 2024.

Royal College of Surgeons of England. Preparing for a Consultant Post. Accessed 2026.

7

Less than full time (LTFT) and flexible training in surgery

INTRODUCTION

Flexible working arrangements within the NHS have become an increasingly integral component of modern medical training, offering doctors the opportunity to complete their training programmes in less than full-time (LTFT) hours. This flexible model typically involves working between 50% and 80% of a full-time rota, either as an individual or through job-sharing partnerships. The evolution of LTFT training reflects a growing recognition of the diverse personaland lifestyle factors that influence doctors' ability to maintain a sustainable work-life balance throughout their careers.

Flexibility in training is no longer viewed as an exception but rather as a valued option that supports inclusivity and well-being without compromising educational quality or clinical competence. Whether motivated by caregiving responsibilities, health considerations, or personal development goals, trainees increasingly seek LTFT pathways that accommodate their unique circumstances.

This chapter will explore in detail the eligibility criteria for LTFT working, the formal application and approval processes, and the practical considerations trainees should anticipate. Moreover, it will provide an analysis of the advantages and potential challenges associated with flexible training models. Most importantly, it will offer actionable strategies to maximise learning opportunities and professional growth while working within a reduced hours framework, ensuring that trainees maintain the trajectory towards achieving their full potential as future consultants.

 DOI: 10.1201/9781003537663-7

ELIGIBILITY

All postgraduate doctors in training, including those enrolled in academic programmes, are eligible to apply for LTFT working arrangements. Applications can be made either at the point of entry into training or at any stage during the training programme once accepted.

The decision to pursue flexible working is often motivated by a range of personal and professional circumstances. Trainees may seek LTFT hours to achieve a better work-life balance, manage caregiving responsibilities, or accommodate health needs. Additionally, some doctors maintain commitments beyond clinical medicine, such as involvement in national or international competitive sports, leadership roles, research activities, or religious and non-medical pursuits, and therefore may require flexibility to allocate their time effectively.

It is strongly advised that trainees considering LTFT working engage in open discussions with their Assigned Educational Supervisor (AES) and Training Programme Director (TPD) to explore how flexible working might best align with their individual circumstances and training requirements. Each application is evaluated on its own merits, taking into account the trainee's unique situation and the demands of their specialty.

Formal applications for LTFT working must be submitted through the appropriate deanery or Local Education and Training Board (LETB), ensuring a structured and transparent approval process.

THE PROCESS FOR APPLYING TO WORK LTFT

Once applicants have obtained in-principle approval from both the AES and the TPD, the next step is to formally apply for LTFT working through the deanery's dedicated online portal. It is important to note that the deanery generally requires a minimum of three months notice to process an LTFT application, so early planning is essential. Following submission, applications will be reviewed and either approved or declined based on eligibility and training needs.

Upon approval, the deanery will formally notify your employing trust of your LTFT status. It is advisable to keep your trust's human resources department informed and engaged throughout the process to ensure seamless coordination and support.

After flexible training arrangements are agreed upon, trainees must liaise with the Joint Committee on Surgical Training (JCST) to confirm that the proposed training timetable aligns with the required curriculum and competency milestones. While TPDs may assist by identifying appropriate posts or suggesting potential slot-share partners, trainees are strongly encouraged to take an active role in securing their own slot-share partner. Leveraging professional networks, prior contacts, or seeking assistance from the TPD can facilitate this process.

It is important to highlight that once LTFT working is approved, reapplication is not necessary at the start of each new rotation. However, trainees must communicate directly with each host placement in advance to agree on their specific work schedule, ensuring clarity and mutual understanding before commencing each placement.

IMPACT ON TRAINING AND EXPECTED CERTIFICATE OF COMPLETION OF TRAINING (CCT)

Although LTFT working reduces the number of hours trainees spend in clinical practice, it does not alter the fundamental requirements for progression set by the JCST. Trainees must still achieve all prescribed competencies to progress successfully through their training.

The principal challenge for LTFT trainees lies in the reduced clinical contact time, which may extend the timeframe needed to acquire essential skills and competencies. Consequently, those who remain in LTFT status for the entirety of their training should anticipate a potentially longer training period before achieving their CCT, with a possible delay in advancement to consultant-level positions.

MAXIMISING EDUCATIONAL OPPORTUNITIES WHILE WORKING LTFT

One of the greatest hurdles for LTFT trainees is ensuring sufficient exposure to clinical learning experiences within the constraints of limited working hours. To overcome this, trainees must adopt a proactive and strategic approach to time management.

With guidance from their TPD and AES, LTFT trainees should carefully structure their schedules to ensure equitable access to a balanced range of educational activities, including outpatient clinics, theatre sessions, and deanery-led teaching programmes. Keeping detailed records of all training opportunities, including work-based assessments, is essential for monitoring progress and demonstrating competency development.

There may be occasions when valuable educational activities fall on days when LTFT trainees are not scheduled to work. Where feasible, trainees are encouraged to attend these sessions and arrange to take equivalent time off in lieu on alternative working days, ensuring compliance with working time regulations while maximising learning.

By maintaining clear communication with supervisors and taking ownership of their training journey, LTFT trainees can successfully navigate the challenges of reduced hours without compromising the quality of their professional development.

The following table provides a summary of the key advantages and potential drawbacks of working LTFT.

Advantages of working LTFT	Disadvantages of working LTFT
• Better work-life balance – more time with family/loved ones/friends, reduced fatigue and greater focus.	• Lower take-home pay and wages due to reduced working hours.
• Opportunities to pursue additional interests outside of medicine – enables development of alternative careers and personal growths.	• Longer training period – takes longer to achieve competencies and skills.
• Reduction in membership fees – significant reductions and cost-savings.	• Reduced contact time and lack of continuity of care for patients.
• Can return to full-time work at any stage with prior notice.	• Negative perceptions of reduced commitment – may be difficult to integrate into teams due to this bias and negative perceptions.
	• LTFT placements can demand time and effort from programme directors and all those concerned.

KEY RECOMMENDATIONS FOR A SMOOTH TRANSITION TO LTFT TRAINING

- *Identify and Connect with Rota Coordinators Early*: it is essential to determine who manages rota design within your upcoming unit. Establish contact with them well in advance to collaboratively plan a schedule that aligns precisely with your approved LTFT working hours, ensuring compliance and avoiding potential conflicts.
- *Engage Your Trust's LTFT Champion*: each trust appoints an LTFT champion dedicated to supporting trainees working less than full

time. This individual is a valuable resource who can provide guidance, address concerns, and facilitate a positive LTFT experience throughout your training.

- *Leverage Peer Support and Regional Networks*: consider reaching out to current or former LTFT trainees within your region. Their first-hand experiences can offer practical advice and insight. Additionally, professional social media groups and the Royal College of Surgeons England website host a wealth of resources tailored to LTFT trainees, which can be highly beneficial during your transition.

SUMMARY

The uptake of LTFT working is steadily increasing as the medical profession increasingly recognises the importance of work-life balance and well-being. While flexible working offers significant benefits, it also presents unique challenges that necessitate comprehensive support for trainees. Encouraging LTFT trainees to actively engage with educational opportunities and providing them with dedicated guidance from their AES and TPD is essential to their success.

By embracing and promoting flexible working arrangements, the NHS cultivates a more diverse, inclusive, and resilient workforce, one that can effectively navigate the demands of surgical training while maintaining personal well-being. This balance is vital, not only for long-term career satisfaction but also for sustaining excellence in patient care.

BIBLIOGRAPHY

British Medical Association. Less than full-time (LTFT) training guidance for doctors in training. BMA; Accessed 2026. Available at: https://www.bma.org.uk

Health Education England. Less Than Full Time Training Handbook. Version 2, 2021. Made in HEE (HEE North East & Yorkshire). Available at: https://madeinheene.hee.nhs.uk

NHS England. Less Than Full Time Training: National Guidance for Doctors in Training. NHS England; Updated 2023. Available at: https://www.england.nhs.uk

8

Diversity, equity, and the challenge of discrimination in surgery

INTRODUCTION

The National Health Service (NHS) is a microcosm of our society. It carries our shared values and ideals, but also, unavoidably, our imperfections. Although the UK Equality Act (2010) provides comprehensive legal protection against discrimination based on protected characteristics, including race, gender, religion, disability, sexual orientation, and others, inequities continue to persist within many sectors, healthcare included.

Within the NHS and the field of surgery, discrimination may present in both subtle and overt forms. These can range from unconscious bias and microaggressions to explicit exclusionary behaviours or systemic barriers that disadvantage individuals and groups. Such actions not only affect staff well-being, morale, and career progression but can also compromise team dynamics and, ultimately, the quality of patient care.

This chapter will examine the issues of diversity, equity, and inclusion within surgery, exploring how discrimination manifests in the surgical environment, its impact on individuals and institutions, and the collective responsibility to foster a culture of respect, fairness, and belonging across the NHS.

DOI: 10.1201/9781003537663-8

MANAGING DISCRIMINATION FROM PATIENTS AND THEIR RELATIVES

While patients have an unequivocal right to safe and equitable healthcare, healthcare professionals are equally entitled to protection from discriminatory or abusive behaviour. Surgery as a specialty has evolved into a richly diverse field, with surgeons and surgical teams representing a wide spectrum of genders, ethnicities, religions, abilities, and social backgrounds. The expectation is that all patient interactions should be grounded in mutual respect, professionalism, and civility.

Unfortunately, discriminatory behaviour from patients or their relatives does occur. Such behaviour may range from derogatory or prejudiced comments about a clinician's gender, race, religion, or other protected characteristics, to overt hostility including the refusal of care from a particular doctor. According to the 2020 NHS Staff Survey, more than one in four staff members (28.5%) reported experiencing harassment, bullying, or abuse from patients, relatives, or members of the public, and almost one in seven (14.9%) reported physical violence. Racism was the most frequently reported form of discrimination, followed by sexism and intolerance related to religion or sexuality.

The NHS constitution clearly states that patients and the public are expected to treat NHS staff and other patients with respect. It further acknowledges that acts of violence or disturbance on NHS premises may result in prosecution, and that abusive or discriminatory behaviour can lead to restricted access to NHS services. In parallel, the Health and Safety at Work Act 1974 places a legal duty on employers to ensure the health, safety, and welfare of their employees, including protecting them from abuse, bullying, and harassment. Consequently, NHS organisations are obligated to maintain a workplace free from discrimination and bias, upholding a zero-tolerance policy towards any form of abuse or prejudice.

Employers must provide clear mechanisms for reporting, investigating, and addressing incidents of discrimination from patients or their relatives. Initial responses may include formal warnings, and persistent or severe cases can warrant exclusion from NHS premises or services. Support and debriefing should also be offered to affected staff members, ensuring that their well-being is prioritised and that they are supported in deciding how they wish the incident to be managed.

There are, however, situations that warrant a degree of sensitivity and professional judgement. Discriminatory behaviour may occasionally stem from underlying medical or psychiatric conditions such as delirium, dementia, or an acute mental health crisis. Situations involving requests based on clinical appropriateness such as a patient requesting a clinician of a specific gender for intimate examinations or culturally sensitive care must be assessed on a case-by-case basis.

Even in these complex scenarios, inappropriate or discriminatory behaviour should be addressed at an appropriate time to reinforce professional boundaries and maintain mutual respect. Patients and their relatives or legal guardians who display discrimination should be counselled and, where appropriate, asked to apologise. In cases of threat or physical danger, security personnel or the police may need to be involved to safeguard staff.

Ultimately, recognising and addressing discrimination from patients and relatives is essential to preserving a safe, respectful, and inclusive working environment. Surgical teams must feel supported, empowered to report incidents, and confident that action will be taken. By doing so, the NHS not only fulfils its legal and moral obligations but also models the values of equity and respect that underpin the practice of medicine itself.

ADDRESSING DISCRIMINATION WITHIN THE SURGICAL PROFESSION

There is a widely acknowledged concern that a culture of discrimination and bullying remains deeply rooted within the surgical profession. In 2021, the Royal College of Surgeons of England commissioned an independent review, led by Baroness Helena Kennedy KC, to examine issues surrounding diversity, inclusion, and belonging in surgery. This initiative followed increasing reports, particularly from women and people of colour, who spoke out about their longstanding experiences of bias and exclusion.

The findings of the resulting report were both revealing and sobering, exposing persistent inequities and systemic barriers within the profession. Key conclusions highlighted that women continue to face sexism and harassment at alarming rates; Black and minority ethnic (BME) doctors experience slower career progression and are disproportionately represented in non-training roles and many perceive the College as unreflective of their backgrounds and experiences. The report also noted that BME doctors are more frequently referred to regulatory bodies, that socioeconomic background influences medical students' decisions to apply for surgical training, and that leadership positions remain overwhelmingly dominated by white men.

Through personal testimonies, the report shed light on the ongoing challenges faced by women, BME surgeons, members of the LGBTQ+ community, and those living with disabilities, often driven by conscious or unconscious bias. These issues not only inflict harm on individuals but also undermine team cohesion, productivity, and the overall effectiveness of the NHS. The consequences are far-reaching, including increased absenteeism, higher staff turnover, and reduced quality of patient care.

In response, the Royal College of Surgeons pledged to take decisive action to foster a culture that is inclusive, equitable, and respectful. Its commitment is clear: to be an organisation that embodies fairness and anti-discrimination, upholding the highest professional and surgical standards, and promoting the best outcomes for patients through respect and compassion for patients and colleagues alike.

To realise this vision, the review set out sixteen recommendations. These included ensuring that the College Council reflects the diversity of its membership, implementing anti-discriminatory policies in recruitment and selection, and amplifying the voices of underrepresented groups such as Women in Surgery, Parents in Surgery, locally employed surgeons, LGBTQ+ surgeons, and those with disabilities. Further recommendations focussed on addressing differential attainment in surgical examinations, creating fellowships dedicated to diversity, equity and inclusion, expanding mentoring programmes for those from marginalised backgrounds, and diversifying the pipeline of medical students entering surgical training.

By commissioning and publishing this review, the Royal College of Surgeons demonstrated both courage and accountability in confronting discrimination within its ranks. Through the comprehensive recommendations that followed, the College has signalled its determination to champion diversity, model inclusive leadership, and drive meaningful change within the surgical community and across the wider NHS.

CONCLUSION

Addressing discrimination and bias within surgery and the wider NHS requires a sustained, multi-faceted approach. Meaningful progress depends on more than policy statements: it demands genuine cultural transformation built on accountability, education, and inclusive leadership.

Awareness and training programmes must foster an understanding of unconscious bias and empower staff to challenge discrimination with confidence. Robust policies and transparent systems of accountability are equally vital to ensure fairness and trust across the profession.

Leaders play a central role in shaping this change by embedding diversity, equity, and compassion into every aspect of organisational practice. Creating a culture where all professionals feel valued and supported not only improves staff well-being but also enhances teamwork, clinical performance, and patient outcomes.

Ultimately, equity in the surgical profession is not only a moral imperative but a clinical necessity. By working collectively to promote respect and inclusivity, we can build a healthcare system where every clinician can thrive and every patient receives the highest standard of compassionate, equitable care.

BIBLIOGRAPHY

How to manage discrimination from patients and their guardians/relatives (2022) BMA Guidance. Available at: https://www.bma.org.uk/media/5144/bma-guidance-on-how-to-deal-with-discrimination-from-patients-march-2022.pdf

NHS constitution for england - gov.uk (2012) NHS Constitution. Available at: https://www.gov.uk/government/publications/the-nhs-constitution-for-england

NHS England. NHS staff morale improves but too many facing abuse (2020) NHS England. Available at: https://www.england.nhs.uk/2020/02/nhs-staff-morale-improves-but-too-many-facing-abuse/

9

Challenges in general surgery: Navigating the modern landscape

INTRODUCTION

General surgery today is practised in an environment which is vastly different from that of even a decade ago, and one that continues to evolve. General surgeons must deliver high-quality care amid workforce pressures and inconsistent teams, constrained resources, evolving patient needs and expectations, as well as rapid technological advancements. Alongside these demands lies also a deeper emotional burden of needing to deliver care with compassion in the face of ongoing challenges. This chapter reflects on the key challenges facing general surgeons in this evolving era. It also offers practical, grounded strategies to help surgeons navigate these realities with clarity and purpose, ensuring that, despite the pressures of modern practice, the core commitment to patient-centred care remains unwavering.

THE CHANGING PATIENT DEMOGRAPHIC

Ageing population, multimorbidity, and polypharmacy

General surgeons are increasingly caring for older patients with multiple chronic conditions and frailty. This demographic shift presents significant challenges, as such patients often have complex physiological profiles that increase perioperative risk, prolong recovery, and heighten susceptibility

 DOI: 10.1201/9781003537663-9

to complications, including infection, impaired wound healing, and acute cardiopulmonary events.

Frailty assessment is now a key component of preoperative evaluation. Frailty is linked to reduced physiological reserves and appears to be a stronger predictor of poor outcomes (delirium, longer stays, mortality) than multimorbidity alone in older patients. Many patients with multimorbidity are also frail. Tools such as the Clinical Frailty Scale (CFS), used alongside validated risk stratification instruments, including ACS NSQIP (American College of Surgeons' National Surgical Quality Improvement Program) and P-POSSUM (Physiological and Perioperative Severity Score for the enumeration of Morbidity and Mortality), can help identify patients at increased risk of post-operative complications, prolonged hospital stay, and mortality. These assessments support informed decision-making and enable tailored care pathways to improve recovery.

Ageing populations also have a higher prevalence of chronic multisystem disease, including diabetes and insulin resistance, cardiovascular disease, renal impairment, and chronic respiratory conditions, such as asthma and COPD. These comorbidities have a deleterious impact on surgical outcomes, contributing to increased perioperative morbidity, delayed functional recovery, and higher complication rates.

Polypharmacy is common in this patient group and has important perioperative implications. Medications such as immunomodulatory agents may impair wound healing and increase infection risk, while anticoagulants and antiplatelet therapies raise bleeding risk and complicate operative timing and post-operative management. In addition, the ethical challenges of balancing potential surgical benefit against risk and quality of life can be emotionally taxing for surgeons and the wider multidisciplinary team.

Managing older and frail patients requires a holistic, multidisciplinary approach. This care is often resource- and time-intensive, requiring extended pre- and post-operative planning and coordination across multiple teams and disciplines.

THE CHANGING DISEASE PROFILE

Obesity, chronic diseases, and mental health conditions

Rates of obesity among both adults and children continue to rise globally, presenting increasing challenges for surgical care. In England, approximately 29% of adults are classified as obese. Among children, around one in ten aged 4–5 years are obese, a figure that increases to approximately one in four among those aged 10–11 years. Obesity not only increases the technical complexity of surgical procedures but also significantly elevates operative risk, including infection, cardiovascular strain, respiratory compromise, and thromboembolic disease. Furthermore, obesity-associated comorbidities, such as low-grade systemic inflammation, reduced functional capacity, and type 2 diabetes mellitus, are independent risk factors for impaired wound healing and non-surgical-site infections. In response, surgeons must adapt their operative techniques and collaborate closely with allied healthcare professionals to support preoperative weight optimisation strategies.

In parallel, populations are living longer, often with multiple chronic conditions. Advancing age is associated with an increased prevalence of multisystem disease, including diabetes mellitus, chronic respiratory disease, heart failure, chronic kidney disease, malignancy, and dementia, each of which is known to adversely affect surgical risk. Patients with chronic conditions experience significantly higher rates of post-operative complications and mortality, alongside increased healthcare utilisation and associated costs, placing additional strain on healthcare systems.

The rising prevalence of mental health disorders represents a further and increasingly important challenge. Pre-existing mental health conditions, particularly anxiety, depression, and post-traumatic stress disorder (PTSD), are strongly associated with poorer surgical outcomes across a range of specialties. Depression and anxiety are linked to more severe and prolonged post-operative pain, while chronic stress and anxiety contribute to sustained elevations in cortisol and inflammatory markers, impairing immune function and delaying wound healing. Overall, patients with pre-existing mental health conditions tend to experience prolonged recovery, higher complication rates, and increased healthcare utilisation. Accordingly, the integration of mental health assessment and support into surgical care pathways is essential to optimise outcomes and enhance patient experience.

RISING DEMAND AND PATIENT EXPECTATIONS

Rising demand within the NHS is largely driven by demographic change and the increasing complexity of patients' healthcare needs. An ageing population, combined with a growing prevalence of chronic and multimorbid conditions, has substantially increased demand for surgical and perioperative services. In addition, persistent healthcare inequalities mean that individuals from lower socioeconomic backgrounds and those living in more deprived areas often develop long-term conditions at an earlier age. This contributes to greater cumulative healthcare utilisation, higher expenditure, and increased pressure on already stretched services.

At the same time, patient expectations of healthcare are evolving. Influenced in part by access to digital and consumer-oriented services, patients now expect more personalised care. Greater access to online health information has also resulted in patients being more informed and actively engaged in their treatment. Consequently, there is an increasing expectation of shared decision-making, with patients wishing to understand their options and to have their values and preferences incorporated into care planning.

The convergence of rising demand and heightened patient expectations has placed significant strain on the healthcare system. Workforce shortages have intensified as demand continues to outpace existing resources, contributing to service pressures across surgical pathways. In response to these challenges, surgeons must not only continue to deliver high-quality care but also refine their communication skills in a transparent, patient-centred approach. Aligning treatment plans with patient values through effective shared decision-making is essential to maintaining trust and within a resource-constrained environment.

FUNDING AND RESOURCE MANAGEMENT

In resource-limited health systems such as the NHS, surgeons are tasked with maintaining currency in evolving treatments and technologies, while simultaneously balancing the finite resources. The interplay between clinical demand and constrained capacity has significant implications for service delivery, workforce well-being, and patient outcomes.

System pressures and capacity constraints

The 2025 UK Surgical Workforce Census highlights ongoing pressures related to access to operating theatres, staff shortages, and infrastructure limitations. More than half of surgical consultants identified theatre access as a major challenge, driven by insufficient theatre space, lack of theatre staff, and inadequate bed availability, all of which restrict productivity and timely care delivery. Surgeons and trainees frequently work beyond contracted hours to address these gaps, indicating systemic strain rather than isolated local issues. Compounding these issues are maintenance backlogs and ageing facilities that reduce usable capacity. Without reinvestment in estates and equipment, surgical throughput remains constrained, and targets for reducing waiting lists are difficult to achieve, even with substantial workforce commitment.

Resource and equipment gaps

Resource inadequacies extend beyond physical infrastructure to include equipment and supplies necessary for safe surgical care. In some settings, limitations in diagnostic support and critical supplies (e.g. blood products) further challenge service provision. These shortfalls increase operational inefficiencies and necessitate adaptive strategies to prioritise care in the setting of rising demand.

Access to care and wait times

Lengthy wait times for emergency and planned procedures persist as a critical concern. Although the NHS has made incremental progress in reducing waiting lists, backlog pressures remain substantial due to demographic shifts, rising chronic disease prevalence, and the residual impact of the COVID-19 pandemic on service capacity and demand. Waitlist management strategies such as stand-alone elective surgical hubs or ring-fencing surgical beds within hospital Trusts are essential to optimising access within existing constraints.

Evolving technologies

Advancements such as minimally invasive, robotic-assisted, and artificial intelligence (AI)-supported surgical techniques have the potential to improve patient outcomes and efficiency. However, the adoption of these technologies necessitates significant investment in equipment, training, and maintenance. Furthermore, cost-benefit analyses and collaboration with multidisciplinary teams are critical to ensuring safe, equitable, and ethical implementation of these technologies.

Addressing these challenges represents a substantial and complex undertaking, requiring sustained political engagement, long-term commitment, and careful planning by policymakers. Resource allocation must be informed by current and projected clinical demand, while simultaneously accommodating the rapid evolution of healthcare technologies that have the potential to improve efficiency and patient outcomes. Meaningful engagement at a political and policy level is essential to ensure that investment decisions support both service resilience and technological advancement.

Surgeons have an important role to play in this process by contributing to local and regional commissioning groups, where clinical insight can help align funding and service design with population needs.

THE NHS WORKFORCE AND RELATED CHALLENGES

The sustainability of the NHS surgical workforce is under increasing pressure. An ageing consultant workforce, combined with limited theatre access and reduced operative exposure for trainees, threatens future workforce capacity. Approximately 61% of surgical trainees identify theatre access as a key barrier to training, highlighting the need for proactive workforce planning. Strategies such as the development of surgical hubs with protected training time, greater use of simulation, structured mentorship, and alignment of training numbers with projected service demand are essential. The expansion of multidisciplinary teams, including physician associates, has the potential to improve service delivery; however, clear role delineation and robust supervision are required to ensure that surgical training and patient safety are not compromised.

Ongoing trends towards subspecialisation and centralisation have improved outcomes for complex care but risk diminishing generalist expertise and reducing local access. Training models must therefore balance core general surgical competencies with subspecialist development, while policy decisions should consider geographical access and patient preference alongside outcomes.

Medico-legal pressures continue to drive defensive practice, increasing costs and unnecessary investigations. Strengthened clinical governance and education on medico-legal standards can help mitigate these effects.

Burnout remains prevalent among surgeons, with 30%–60% reporting symptoms related to workload, responsibility, and emotional strain. Institutional support for well-being, optimised job planning, and normalising access to mental health services are critical. Surgeons also face occupational health risks, particularly musculoskeletal injury, underscoring the importance of ergonomic training and equipment. Finally, persistent gender and ethnic disparities in surgical training and leadership highlight the need for sustained efforts to improve diversity and inclusion through targeted recruitment, mentorship, and flexible training pathways.

CONCLUSION

General surgeons today work within an increasingly complex healthcare environment shaped by an ageing population, limited resources, workforce pressures, and rapid technological change. Meeting these challenges requires not only system-level reform but also proactive individual practice and strong collaborative leadership. By grounding clinical work in evidence-based practice, prioritising workforce well-being, advocating for appropriate resource investment, and adopting new technologies in a thoughtful and responsible way, surgeons can continue to deliver high-quality care while protecting their own well-being and job satisfaction.

BIBLIOGRAPHY

British Medical Association. *The Mental Health and Wellbeing of the Medical Workforce*. London: BMA; 2022.

Health Education England. *Surgical Training and the Future Workforce*. London: HEE; 2023.

Hsu CY, Prasad KDV, Abbas Al-Khafaji ZK, Saidov J, Naeim M. Mental Health and Surgery: Integrating Psychological Care into Surgical Treatment Plans: Letter to Editor. *International Journal of Surgery*. 2025 Sep; 111(9):6482–6485.

Josephs CA, Shaffer VO, Kucera WB. Impact of Mental Health on General Surgery Patients and Strategies to Improve Outcomes. *The American Surgeon*. 2023 Jun; 89(6):2636–2643.

NHS England. *Elective Recovery Plan*. London: NHS England; 2023.

NHS England. *Annual Report and Accounts 2024–25*. London: NHS England; 2025. Available from: UK Government publications.

NHS Workforce Race Equality Standard (WRES). *2023 Data Analysis Report*. London: NHS England; 2024.

Plassmeier L, Hankir MK, Seyfried F. Impact of Excess Body Weight on Postsurgical Complications. *Visceral Medicine*. 2021 Aug; 37(4): 287–297.

Podmore B, Hutchings A, van der Meulen J, Aggarwal A, Konan S. Impact of Comorbid Conditions on Outcomes of Hip and Knee Replacement Surgery: A Systematic Review and Meta-analysis. *BMJ Open*. 2018 Jul 11; 8(7):e021784.

Rosen CB, Roberts SE, Wirtalla CJ, Ramadan OI, Keele LJ, Kaufman EJ, Halpern SD, Kelz RR. Analyzing Impact of Multimorbidity on Long-Term Outcomes after Emergency General Surgery: A Retrospective Observational Cohort Study. *Journal of the American College of Surgeons*. 2022 Nov 1; 235(5):724–735.

RCS England. *Protecting Surgical Training: Standards and Recommendations*. London: RCS England; 2022.

RCS of England. *Physician Associates in Surgery: Guidance for Employers and Surgeons*. London: RCS England; 2023.

RCS of England. *UK Surgical Workforce Census 2025*. London: RCS England; 2025. Available from: Royal College of Surgeons of England website.

Shanafelt TD, Balch CM, Bechamps G, et al. Burnout and Career Satisfaction among American Surgeons. *Annals of Surgery*. 2009; 250(3):463–471.

Swarbrick CJ; SNAP-3 collaborators; Williams K, Evans B, Blake HA, Poulton T, Nava S, Shah A, Martin P, Partridge JSL, Moppett IK. Postoperative Outcomes in Older Patients Living with Frailty and Multimorbidity in the UK: SNAP-3, a Snapshot Observational Study. *British Journal of Anaesthesia*. 2025 Jul; 135(1):166–176.

UK Department of Health and Social Care. *Innovation and New Technology to Help Reduce NHS Waiting Lists*. London: DHSC; 2023. Available from: UK Government website.

West CP, Dyrbye LN, Shanafelt TD. Physician Burnout: Contributors, Consequences and Solutions. *Journal of Internal Medicine*. 2018; 283(6):516–529.

10

What to do when things don't go as planned

INTRODUCTION

Surgery is among the most demanding of medical disciplines that requires sustained commitment over many years. Yet, despite best intentions and considerable effort, not every trainee completes the journey as originally envisioned. It is not uncommon, at various stages of training, to experience uncertainty about one's chosen path. For some, these doubts are transient and manageable; for others, disillusionment and discouragement may gradually set in.

The intricate, multistage nature of surgical training inevitably presents a series of challenges: academic, technical, and personal. These challenges may, at times, feel insurmountable. Feelings of inadequacy, frustration, or diminished motivation can emerge, particularly when progress stalls or when comparisons with peers heighten self-doubt. Moreover, unforeseen circumstances, be they personal issues, family responsibilities, or other life events, can unexpectedly disrupt even the most carefully laid plans.

When the trajectory of one's career diverges from expectations, it can be a profoundly unsettling experience. The sense of uncertainty that follows can erode confidence and purpose. Attempting to persevere in isolation, without adequate support or mentorship, risks compounding the strain and may ultimately lead to stress, disengagement, or burnout.

This chapter seeks to provide perspective and guidance for those navigating such turning points. It will explore ways in which the aspiring surgeon can take stock of their situation, re-evaluate their goals, and manage setbacks with compassion, clarity, and professionalism, ultimately enabling them to find renewed direction, whether within surgery or along an alternative, fulfilling path.

DOI: 10.1201/9781003537663-10

FIRST STEPS IN REGAINING CONTROL

When the trajectory of your surgical training no longer aligns with your expectations, it can be disorienting and distressing. The first and most important step towards regaining control is to pause, take a deliberate breath, and begin to understand the situation with clarity and honesty. Rather than reacting impulsively or allowing frustration to dictate your decisions, it is vital to approach the moment with composure and curiosity.

If circumstances allow, take some annual leave to create space for rest and clear reflection. Begin by engaging in structured self-reflection. The goal is not self-criticism, but insight and an opportunity to discern the underlying factors contributing to your current difficulties. Consider the following questions and respond to them as candidly as possible:

- Why do I feel my surgical career is not progressing as expected?
- Are there limited opportunities for advancement or professional growth within my current environment?
- Have personal challenges such as health, relationships, or family responsibilities begun to affect my training or performance?
- Are there workplace issues, such as team dynamics, supervision, or institutional culture, that are hindering my development?
- Have my interests or professional aspirations evolved since I began training?
- Is there another role or specialty that now feels more aligned with my skills, values, or passions?
- Am I experiencing fatigue, demotivation, or early signs of burnout as a result of sustained pressure or unmet expectations?

Engaging deeply with these questions helps to shift the narrative from helplessness to understanding. Clarity about why you are struggling enables you to begin planning how to move forward, whether that involves seeking mentorship, adjusting your goals, or exploring new directions within or beyond surgery.

ACTIONS AND CONSIDERATIONS WHEN THINGS DON'T GO AS PLANNED

Reaching a point in your surgical career where progress feels uncertain can be deeply unsettling. Yet, this juncture can also become a pivotal opportunity for reflection, recalibration, and growth. The steps you take now will help determine how effectively you regain direction and purpose.

The following considerations are intended to support you as you navigate this phase with professionalism, self-awareness, and compassion.

Seek guidance from mentors and trusted colleagues

Mentorship is an invaluable source of perspective during periods of uncertainty. Engage openly with your supervisors, mentors, and trusted colleagues within the profession. Their insights, often shaped by personal experience, can illuminate potential solutions, identify opportunities for growth, and provide reassurance that challenges such as yours are not uncommon. Experienced mentors can also help you identify practical steps to address the factors contributing to your situation, whether they are technical, interpersonal, or systemic.

Consult career advisors with expertise in medicine or surgery

Professional career advisors, particularly those specialising in medicine, can provide structured guidance to help you explore your options and set achievable goals. They can assist in clarifying your strengths, identifying alternative career paths, and developing strategies for overcoming professional obstacles. Most NHS trusts, deaneries, and professional bodies such as the BMA offer access to such advisory services. You may also choose to connect with independent medical career coaches through professional networks such as LinkedIn. Engaging in a few targeted sessions can help you view your situation from a broader, more objective perspective.

Draw on the support of family and friends

Family members and close friends often bring an understanding of your personal values, character, and life circumstances that professional contacts may not. They can offer emotional support and candid perspectives, helping you to rediscover confidence and balance. However, it is important to recognise the potential limitations of their advice. While their intentions are well-meaning, they may lack the contextual understanding of surgical training and its unique demands. Use these conversations as a means of gaining personal clarity and emotional grounding, rather than as the sole basis for professional decision-making.

Connect with peers who have faced similar challenges

Speaking with other surgeons who have experienced comparable difficulties can be immensely reassuring and constructive. Whether through formal networks, professional associations, or informal connections, sharing experiences helps normalise the challenges of surgical training and alleviates feelings of isolation. Learning how others have navigated similar turning points can offer both inspiration and practical strategies to guide your next steps.

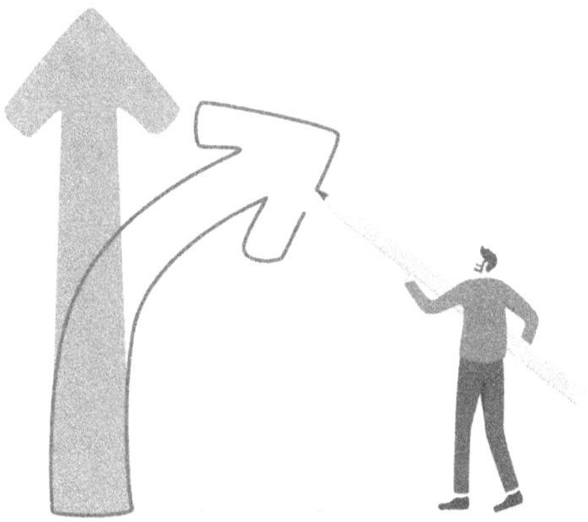

Explore alternative paths within medicine

Medicine is a broad and evolving profession, and the skills developed through surgical training such as precision, problem-solving, teamwork, and resilience are highly transferable. If you find that surgery no longer aligns with your aspirations or circumstances, consider other specialties that allow you to leverage your expertise while accommodating different priorities.

Some former trainees find fulfilment in fields such as radiology, where procedural and anatomical knowledge are still central but work-life balance may be improved. Others transition into emergency medicine, sports medicine, or aesthetic medicine, applying surgical dexterity in new contexts.

Beyond clinical practice, rewarding opportunities exist in medical education, research, medical journalism, career coaching, medical law, and industry consulting with organisations such as pharmaceutical or device companies. Attending specialty-specific conferences, career fairs, and networking events can serve as valuable entry points for exploring these avenues.

Consider career options beyond medicine

For some, stepping entirely outside the field of medicine may represent the most authentic and fulfilling choice. While less common, such transitions are increasingly recognised as legitimate and successful pathways. Surgeons are highly employable in a variety of sectors due to their analytical thinking, leadership, and problem-solving abilities.

Potential alternatives include roles in public health policy, or civil service positions within the Department of Health and Social Care, where medical graduates are often sought for graduate fast-track programmes. Others have embraced entrepreneurship, so-called "doctorpreneurship," creating start-ups or ventures across diverse industries. Exploring these routes often begins by attending multidisciplinary conferences, engaging with professional networks, and seeking mentorship from individuals who have made similar transitions.

Leaving medicine, whether temporarily or permanently, should not be viewed as failure. Rather, it can be an act of self-preservation and purposeful reinvention, an opportunity to align your work with your evolving values and aspirations.

Take time to pause and reflect

Sometimes, the most constructive action is to take a deliberate break. The stigma surrounding career breaks in medicine is diminishing, and more doctors are recognising the value of stepping back to prioritise well-being and clarity. If you are feeling depleted, demotivated, or burnt out, a structured period of leave can provide essential time to rest and reassess your goals.

During this period, allow yourself the space to explore questions such as the following:

- Which aspects of medicine energise me, and which deplete me?
- Am I seeking a different pace, focus, or balance in my professional life?
- What skills or passions might I want to develop further?

A career break can also serve as an opportunity to travel, volunteer, pursue further study, or gain experience in a new field. Many doctors return from such breaks with renewed perspective, improved mental health, and a clearer sense of purpose. Whether the outcome is a recommitment to surgery or a new direction altogether, the process of pausing and reflecting is an essential investment in your long-term well-being and professional fulfilment.

CONCLUSIONS

It is essential not to let the time and effort you have already invested in surgical training deter you from making a change if the path no longer feels right for you. Every stage of your journey contributes to your growth, regardless of the ultimate direction it takes.

Equally important is granting yourself permission to pause. Taking a brief, restorative break can create the mental space needed to reflect objectively, regain perspective, and reconnect with what truly drives you. This period of reflection often brings clarity that is difficult to achieve amid the intensity of day-to-day clinical work.

Remember, stepping back to reassess your direction is not a sign of weakness or failure. On the contrary, it reflects maturity, insight, and professional self-awareness. It represents the first step towards a more deliberate, balanced, and compassionate approach to your career, one grounded in authenticity and personal fulfilment.

BIBLIOGRAPHY

https://medicfootprints.org/alternative-careers-for-doctors-the-ultimate-list/

https://resources.nejmcareercenter.org/article/outside-the-fold-exploring-nonclinical-work-opportunities-for-physicians/

11

Expanding horizons: Alternative and portfolio careers in surgery

INTRODUCTION

While traditional surgical careers focus primarily on clinical practice, an increasing number of surgeons are pursuing careers that combine operative work with other professional interests. This cultural change of balancing a surgeon's special interests in addition to their traditional surgical careers can result in a rewarding and fulfilling career. The emergence of portfolio careers and growing appeal of flexible and multidisciplinary roles reflect this evolving professional landscape.

This chapter will explore alternative and portfolio careers in greater depth, outlining opportunities where surgeons can make significant contributions including in academic surgery, education, leadership roles, technology and innovation, medical writing, law and humanitarian work. These roles may be in line with existing surgical or clinical practice, or in alternative fields altogether.

If a surgeon would like to explore diversification in their careers, there are many resources online and offline which may help. Speaking to colleagues who have portfolio careers you have an interest in is often useful – offering to shadow or work with them can be illuminating to share experiences and learn how to enter these careers. The following portfolio careers are only a limited range of examples – it is often useful to network and explore the options available.

DOI: 10.1201/9781003537663-11

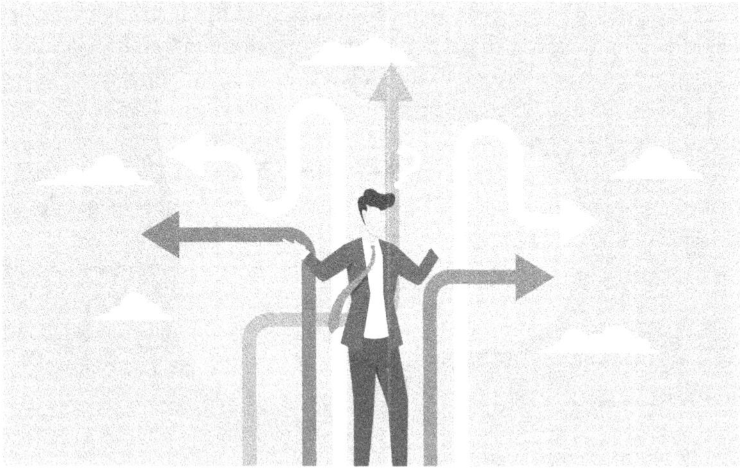

Academic and teaching careers

Research is a fundamental and highly valued component of surgical training, offering surgeons unique opportunities to advance both their clinical expertise and the broader field of medicine. Pursuing an academic career in surgery requires a strong commitment to scholarly endeavours while maintaining the highest clinical standards. Although there is no single defined pathway, trainees are often encouraged to seek competitive academic training posts. Early stage opportunities include the Academic Foundation Programme (AFP) route during the foundation years, while more advanced trainees may pursue Academic Clinical Fellowships (ACF) within core or higher specialty training. These posts typically align with the National Institute for Health and Care Research (NIHR) clinical academic pathway, providing structured support to develop research skills alongside clinical training through protected research time.

As surgeons progress, they may also apply for Clinical Lecturer positions, which combine research and teaching responsibilities within university-affiliated hospitals. These roles provide a platform for contributing to the education of medical students and junior trainees, fostering the next generation of surgical talent while advancing one's own academic portfolio.

It is important to note that these academic pathways are not prerequisite for those aspiring to have fulfilling academic careers in surgery.

Pursuit of higher degrees, such as a master's or PhD, is strongly encouraged for those seeking to deepen their research expertise. Trainees may apply for out-of-programme research experiences to undertake these degrees, as the intensity and time commitment of formal research often necessitate a temporary pause in clinical training. These experiences not only enhance research capabilities but also develop skills in scientific writing, grant applications, and teaching, which are invaluable for a long-term academic career in surgery.

Others take on clinical leadership positions, or roles in commissioning bodies and the more nascent integrated care systems, and others train in and develop teaching and mentoring skills as GP trainers, educators, and appraisers. There are a multitude of options as outlined in the flowchart on the next page.

LEADERSHIP CAREERS

Surgeons are uniquely positioned to excel in leadership and management roles across healthcare trusts, regional or national bodies, and governmental organisations. The skills developed through surgical practice such as decisive leadership, critical-thinking and clear communication translate seamlessly into high-level leadership settings.

Pursuing formal leadership development, such as a master's in business administration (MBA), or gaining experience in leadership roles both within and beyond medicine, can be highly valuable when preparing for these positions. Engaging in these opportunities not only enhances administrative and strategic capabilities but also enables surgeons to influence healthcare delivery, drive innovation, and lead multidisciplinary teams with confidence and impact.

CAREERS IN TECHNOLOGY AND INNOVATION

Careers at the intersection of medicine, technology, and innovation offer surgeons and healthcare professionals the opportunity to shape the future of patient care. Advances in surgical technologies including robotics, digital health, artificial intelligence, and data analytics are transforming clinical practice, and clinicians with surgical expertise bring invaluable insights to the design and implementation of these innovations. Surgeons may choose new career paths in technology-driven roles, whether through collaborations with industry or start-ups. Skills in project management, interdisciplinary collaboration, and digital literacy, combined with clinical experience, are highly sought-after, and make applicants form a surgical background highly favoured.

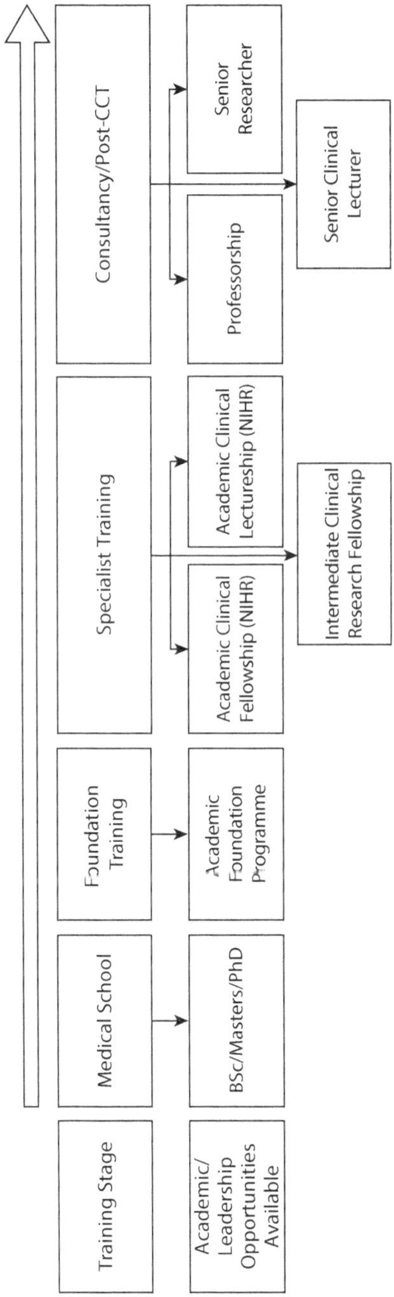

Training Stage
Academic/ Leadership Opportunities Available
Medical School
BSc/Masters/PhD
Foundation Training
Academic Foundation Programme
Specialist Training
Academic Clinical Fellowship (NIHR)
Academic Clinical Lectureship (NIHR)
Intermediate Clinical Research Fellowship
Consultancy/Post-CCT
Professorship
Senior Researcher
Senior Clinical Lecturer

CAREERS IN MEDICAL WRITING

Medical writing offers surgeons a unique avenue to combine clinical expertise with communication and knowledge dissemination. This career pathway includes a variety of activities, such as preparing and editing scientific manuscripts, contributing educational or reflective articles to medical journals, and authoring books. Surgeons bring invaluable insight to medical writing, ensuring accuracy, clarity, and relevance in clinical and scientific material. Medical writing not only provides an enjoyable and intellectually stimulating career path but also allows surgeons to influence the way medical knowledge is shared, improving patient care and advancing the field beyond the operating room.

CAREERS IN MEDICO-LEGAL FIELDS

Medico-legal work provides doctors with the opportunity to apply their clinical expertise in legal and regulatory contexts. Clinicians may become involved in activities such as providing expert witness testimony, preparing medico-legal reports, advising on clinical negligence cases, or contributing to policy and regulatory reviews. This work requires a thorough understanding of both medical standards and legal frameworks, along with strong analytical and communication skills. Pursuing medico-legal work alongside clinical commitments allows doctors to diversify their professional portfolio, develop additional income streams, and gain insight into the legal aspects of healthcare.

HUMANITARIAN WORK AND GLOBAL SURGERY AS A PORTFOLIO CAREER

According to the latest figures from the World Health Organization (WHO), approximately two-thirds of the world's population do not have access to safe, effective, and affordable surgery. Humanitarian work and global surgery offer surgeons the opportunity to apply their skills in resource-limited settings, addressing the wide disparities that exist in surgical care across the globe, and making a tangible impact on vulnerable populations. Many surgeons engage with UK-based charitable organisations such as Operation International UK or Operation Hernia, contributing to surgical missions, training local healthcare teams, and supporting capacity-building initiatives. On a broader scale, international organisations like Médecins Sans Frontières (Doctors Without Borders) provide opportunities to deliver surgical care in conflict zones, disaster-affected areas, and underserved regions worldwide.

Pursuing humanitarian surgery as part of a portfolio career allows clinicians to maintain their NHS or private practice while dedicating time to global initiatives, medical education, and capacity development. This pathway develops skills in adaptability, cross-cultural communication, and leadership, while offering a deeply rewarding professional experience. Surgeons involved in global health also have the opportunity to influence policy, advocate for equitable healthcare access, and contribute to research in global surgery, blending clinical expertise with social impact.

CONCLUSION

Portfolio careers in surgery offer an exceptional breadth of opportunities, allowing surgeons to tailor their professional lives to their individual interests, skills, and values. Whether through research, teaching, leadership, humanitarian work, technology, medico-legal practice, or medical writing, there is vast scope to combine clinical excellence with diverse and fulfilling pursuits. This variety not only provides personal satisfaction and enjoyment but also enhances professional growth by developing a wide array of transferable skills. Engaging in a portfolio career enriches both the surgeon and the wider healthcare community, fostering a more adaptable, reflective, and well-rounded professional capable of contributing meaningfully within and beyond the operating theatre.

BIBLIOGRAPHY

BCG. Medical candidates | BCG [Internet]. BCG. 2024 [cited 2024 Nov 12]. Available from: https://careers.bcg.com/global/en/students/medical-candidates

Dichoso E. Alternative careers for doctors: The ultimate list [Internet]. *Medic Footprints*. 2024 [cited 2024 Nov 12]. Available from: https://medicfootprints.org/alternative-careers-for-doctors-the-ultimate-list/

Health Education Northwest. Resources for doctors who are considering leaving medicine [Internet]. [cited 2024 Nov 12]. Available from: https://www.nwpgmd.nhs.uk/sites/default/files/Resources%20for%20doctors%20who%20are%20considering%20leaving%20medicinepdf.pdf

http://medicalsuccess.net/

https://www.bma.org.uk/careers/careers_service/index.jsp

Life After Medicine. Life after medicine [Internet]. Lifeaftermedicine.co.uk. 2024 [cited 2024 Nov 12]. Available from: http://www.lifeaftermedicine.co.uk/

McKinsey. McKinsey's UK Medical Elective Programme | United Kingdom | McKinsey & Company [Internet]. www.mckinsey.com. Available from: https://www.mckinsey.com/uk/careers/uk-medical-elective-programme

Medic Footprints. Medic Footprints | The doctors' alternative & diverse careers platform [Internet]. Medic Footprints. Available from: https://medicfootprints.org/

Surgical health policy 2025–35: strengthening essential services for tomorrow's needs. *Health Policy*. 2025 August 23; 406(10505): P860–880.

University of Nottingham. Alternative career choices - The University of Nottingham [Internet]. Nottingham.ac.uk. 2024 [cited 2024 Nov 12]. Available from: https://www.nottingham.ac.uk/careers/students/graduatejobs/career-paths/medicine/alternative.aspx

12

Emotional survival in surgery

INTRODUCTION

Surgery is one of the most physically and mentally demanding professions within medicine. The pursuit of surgical excellence often comes at the cost of personal and professional sacrifices that can overtime impact well-being and health. Long and unpredictable working hours, demanding on-call schedules, and additional commitments to research, teaching, and administrative duties can cumulatively lead to chronic physical fatigue and emotional exhaustion. The COVID-19 global pandemic has further highlighted the critical importance of safeguarding both physical and mental health within the surgical profession. This chapter will explore the importance of safeguarding mental and emotional health for career longevity and productivity.

EMOTIONAL CHALLENGES ENCOUNTERED THROUGHOUT A SURGICAL CAREER

Surgeons operate within a uniquely demanding professional environment and, as a result, may encounter a wide range of emotional difficulties over the course of their careers. These challenges arise from the inherent pressures of surgical practice, organisational and cultural factors, and personal circumstances, often interacting in complex ways.

CHRONIC STRESS AND EMOTIONAL STRAIN

Day-to-day stress is an almost universal feature of surgical practice. Surgeons routinely work in high-stakes environments that require rapid

DOI: 10.1201/9781003537663-12

decision-making, often with life-or-death consequences. Procedural complexity, increasingly complex patient co-morbidities, and the frequent mismatch between clinical demand and available resources contribute to sustained emotional pressure. Heavy workloads, long working hours, night shifts, fatigue, and sleep deprivation can impair both cognitive function and emotional resilience. In addition, administrative burdens and inefficiencies within healthcare systems such as delays, poorly designed pathways, and staffing shortages add further layers of frustration and stress to daily practice.

DEPRESSION AND ANXIETY

Rates of depression and anxiety among surgeons are rising, reflecting both personal and work-related stressors. Difficulties in maintaining a healthy work-life balance, relationship or family pressures, and individual personality traits such as perfectionism and excessive self-criticism can increase vulnerability. Work-related factors, including bullying, harassment, inadequate organisational support, limited access to well-being resources, and a perceived lack of recognition or reward for clinical work, further exacerbate psychological distress. Left unaddressed, these conditions can impair performance, job satisfaction, and overall quality of life.

PROFESSIONAL ISOLATION

Although surgery is inherently team-based, elements of a surgical career can be isolating. Rotational training, working in unfamiliar environments, and relocation away from established support networks can contribute to a sense of disconnection. Experiences of bias, discrimination, or prejudice may further compound feelings of isolation, particularly for individuals who feel marginalised or "othered" within their workplace. This isolation can limit opportunities for informal peer support and increase emotional vulnerability.

BURNOUT: DEFINITION, PREVALENCE, AND IMPACT

Burnout, defined as a state of emotional exhaustion, depersonalisation, and reduced personal accomplishment resulting from prolonged workplace stress, has emerged as a major concern within surgery. Its effects are far-reaching and can influence behaviour, decision-making, and responses to error. The widely described "burnout epidemic" undermines professional fulfilment and has been linked to poorer team dynamics, reduced empathy, increased error rates, and compromised patient safety. Among medical specialties, surgery consistently reports some of the highest burnout rates, reflecting its intense workload and the gravity of clinical responsibility.

Multiple factors contribute to burnout, including frequent night shifts, excessive weekly working hours, balancing work with parental or care responsibilities, and the pressures associated with certain subspecialties. Importantly, many surgeons fail to recognise early warning signs, seeking help only once symptoms have become entrenched.

Education and self-awareness are therefore critical in preventing and addressing burnout. Evidence-based strategies such as prioritising adequate sleep, maintaining good nutrition and physical activity, taking regular breaks, and moderating alcohol intake can have a meaningful protective effect. While seemingly modest, these measures can interrupt the cycle of exhaustion and emotional depletion that often characterises surgical practice.

PROFESSIONAL DISAPPOINTMENT AND CAREER SETBACKS

Surgeons may also face significant emotional challenges related to disappointment and perceived failure. Not passing postgraduate examinations, failing to secure a desired training post or consultant appointment, or experiencing delayed career progression, often after substantial personal, financial, and emotional investment, can lead to frustration, loss of confidence, and demoralisation.

ADVERSE OUTCOMES, COMPLAINTS, AND REGULATORY SCRUTINY

Managing adverse outcomes and surgical complications is an inevitable part of practice and can provoke profound feelings of guilt, self-doubt, and moral distress. While structured forums such as morbidity and mortality meetings are intended to promote learning, poorly managed discussions may foster cultures of blame rather than reflection. Similarly, dealing with complaints from patients or colleagues can be emotionally taxing and may challenge a surgeon's professional identity.

Referral to, or investigation by, regulatory bodies can be particularly distressing. Beyond the immediate psychological impact, such processes may disrupt careers, damage reputations, and carry the potential for financial strain or loss of professional registration. Litigation further compounds emotional distress, often creating prolonged anxiety, defensive practice, and concerns about career progression.

TOXIC WORKPLACE CULTURES

Finally, toxic workplace cultures characterised by conflict, incivility, bullying, or unprofessional behaviour pose a significant threat to both staff well-being and patient safety. Evidence increasingly demonstrates that poor workplace culture directly impacts communication, team performance, and clinical outcomes, a principle highlighted by the "Civility Saves Lives" campaign. The independent review led by Baroness Kennedy in 2021 reinforced the damaging effects of bullying, harassment, and fear-based cultures within healthcare organisations, emphasising the need for accountability, compassionate leadership, and systemic cultural change.

ADDRESSING EMOTIONAL CHALLENGES AND BUILDING SUPPORTIVE SURGICAL CULTURES

Effectively addressing the emotional challenges encountered throughout a surgical career requires both individual strategies and collective, organisational commitment. Central to this is the creation of cohesive teams and psychologically safe working environments in which surgeons are supported, valued, and able to practise without fear or chronic emotional strain.

MANAGING CHRONIC STRESS AND PREVENTING BURNOUT

Chronic stress is an inherent risk in surgical practice, but its impact can be mitigated through early recognition and proactive management. At an individual level, maintaining physical health through adequate sleep, regular exercise, balanced nutrition, and protected rest periods is fundamental. Equally important is developing self-awareness and recognising early signs of emotional exhaustion, depersonalisation, or reduced professional fulfilment. Time management, realistic goal-setting, and setting boundaries around workload can help limit cumulative stress.

At an organisational level, burnout prevention requires thoughtful job planning, manageable rotas, access to leave, and recognition of the emotional as well as technical demands of surgical work. Education around burnout and well-being should be embedded within training and continuing professional development, normalising discussion of stress and mental health as part of professional competence rather than personal weakness.

BUILDING TEAM COHESION AND PSYCHOLOGICAL SAFETY

High-functioning surgical teams are characterised by trust, mutual respect, and psychological safety where individuals feel able to speak up and raise concerns without fear of blame or reprisal. Leaders play a pivotal role in setting this tone through inclusive behaviour, openness to feedback, and modelling respectful communication. Regular team briefings, debriefings after complex cases, and reflective discussions can strengthen cohesion and shared responsibility.

Psychological safety is particularly important in surgery, where hierarchical structures and performance pressures may otherwise inhibit openness. Cultures that prioritise learning over blame support both patient safety and clinician well-being, allowing teams to address errors, complications, and system failures constructively.

RESPONDING TO TOXIC WORK ENVIRONMENTS

Toxic workplace behaviours, such as bullying, harassment, incivility, or unprofessional conduct, pose serious risks to both staff well-being and patient care. Addressing such environments requires clear institutional policies, robust reporting mechanisms, and visible leadership commitment to behavioural standards. Early intervention, mediation, and accountability are essential to prevent the normalisation of harmful behaviours. Empowering surgeons to raise concerns safely and ensuring appropriate follow-up reinforces trust in organisational processes and reduces fear-driven practice.

COPING WITH ADVERSE OUTCOMES AND COMPLAINTS

Adverse surgical outcomes and complications are an inevitable part of practice and can evoke profound emotional responses, including guilt, shame, and self-doubt. Structured reflective processes, such as well-facilitated morbidity and mortality meetings, should focus on learning and system improvement rather than individual blame. Peer support following adverse events is particularly important, as surgeons may otherwise internalise responsibility and experience isolation.

Similarly, managing patient complaints can be emotionally taxing. Access to mentorship, medico-legal advice, and supportive line management can help surgeons navigate these processes while maintaining perspective and professional confidence.

SUPPORT DURING REGULATORY REFERRALS AND INVESTIGATIONS

Referral to, or investigation by, a regulatory body represents one of the most stressful experiences in a surgical career. Such processes can disrupt professional identity, generate fear regarding reputation and career progression, and cause significant psychological distress. Early access to professional advice, peer support, and mental health services is critical during this period. Organisations should ensure that surgeons undergoing investigation are supported compassionately and fairly, recognising the emotional burden these processes impose.

THE ROLE OF SUPPORT NETWORKS AND FORMAL RESOURCES

Social and professional support networks play a vital role in maintaining emotional resilience. Open conversations with trusted colleagues, friends, or family members can provide perspective and emotional relief. When additional support is required, engagement with general practitioners, occupational health services, or counselling professionals can be instrumental in identifying patterns of stress or burnout and initiating recovery.

A number of professional organisations offer dedicated support for clinicians, including the Royal College of Surgeons (RCS), the Practitioner Health Programme (PHP), the British Medical Association (BMA), and the Doctors' Support Network. These resources provide confidential access to mental health support, advocacy, and guidance tailored to the needs of medical professionals.

REFLECTIVE PRACTICE AND SCHWARTZ ROUNDS

Structured reflective interventions, such as Schwartz Rounds, offer an additional and increasingly valued means of supporting emotional well-being within surgical teams. Schwartz Rounds are multidisciplinary forums that provide a safe, confidential space to explore the emotional and social aspects of healthcare work, focusing on the human experience rather than clinical detail. While long established in psychiatry and medicine, their growing adoption in surgical settings reflects recognition of the emotional impact of high-stakes decision-making, patient loss, and moral distress.

By fostering empathy, shared understanding, and open dialogue, Schwartz Rounds help reduce emotional fatigue, strengthen team cohesion, and counter the culture of emotional suppression that has traditionally characterised surgical practice. Integrating reflective practices into routine clinical life is a powerful strategy for preventing burnout and sustaining long-term mental well-being.

CONCLUSION

Recognising the importance of a surgeon's mental health is essential for fostering a sustainable and effective workforce. Addressing workplace factors such as bullying, harassment, and lack of support can help build a more positive and resilient surgical culture. Creating an environment that values collegiality, open communication, and mutual respect can enhance morale, promote collaboration, and improve overall job satisfaction. Ultimately, surgery is an endurance sport rather than a sprint. Sustaining a long and fulfilling career in this demanding specialty requires stamina, balance, and proactive attention to one's own well-being. If the profession fails to prioritise the physical and mental health of its practitioners, it risks undermining the very foundations upon which surgical excellence is built.

BIBLIOGRAPHY

Bourne T, Wynants L, Peters M, et al. The impact of complaints procedures on the welfare, health and clinical practice of doctors. *BMJ Open*. 2015;5:e006687.

British Medical Association. *The Mental Health and Wellbeing of the Medical Workforce*. London: BMA; 2022.

Doctors' Support Network. *Supporting Doctors with Mental Health Difficulties*. London: Doctors' Support Network; 2022.

Dyrbye LN, Shanafelt TD. Physician burnout: a potential threat to successful health care reform. *Journal of the American Medical Association*. 2011;305(19):2009–2010.

Edmondson AC. Psychological safety and learning behavior in work teams. *Administrative Science Quarterly*. 1999;44(2):350–383.

Edmondson AC. *The Fearless Organization: Creating Psychological Safety in the Workplace for Learning, Innovation, and Growth*. Hoboken, NJ: Wiley; 2018.

Fnais N, Soobiah C, Chen MH, et al. Harassment and discrimination in medical training: a systematic review. *Academic Medicine*. 2014; 89(5):817–827.

General Medical Council. *The State of Medical Education and Practice in the UK*. London: GMC; 2024.

Hall LH, Johnson J, Watt I, Tsipa A, O'Connor DB. Healthcare staff well-being, burnout, and patient safety. *BMJ Open*. 2016;6:e011838.

Kennedy I. *Independent Review into Whistleblowing in the NHS*. London: Department of Health and Social Care; 2021.

Lewis, C. The impact of interprofessional incivility on medical performance, service and patient care: A systematic review. *Future Healthcare Journal*. 2023;10(1), 69–77.

Lown BA, Manning CF. The Schwartz Center Rounds: evaluation of an interdisciplinary approach to enhancing patient-centered communication, teamwork, and provider support. *Academic Medicine*. 2010;85(6):1073–1081.

Maben J, Taylor C, Dawson J, et al. A realist informed mixed-methods evaluation of Schwartz Rounds in England. *Health Services and Delivery Research* 2018;6(37).

Panagioti M, Geraghty K, Johnson J, et al. Association between physician burnout and patient safety, professionalism, and patient satisfaction. *JAMA Internal Medicine*. 2018;178(10):1317–1331.

Practitioner Health Programme. *Annual Report*. London: PHP; 2023.

Royal College of Surgeons of England. *Caring for Surgeons, Caring for Patients*. London: RCS England; 2020.

Shanafelt TD, Balch CM, Bechamps G, et al. Burnout and career satisfaction among American surgeons. *Annals of Surgery*. 2009;250(3):463–471.

Shanafelt TD, Noseworthy JH. Executive leadership and physician well-being: nine organizational strategies to promote engagement and reduce burnout. *Mayo Clinic Proceedings*. 2017;92(1):129–146.

West CP, Dyrbye LN, Shanafelt TD. Physician burnout: contributors, consequences and solutions. *Journal of Internal Medicine*. 2018;283(6):516–529.

Wu AW. Medical error: the second victim. *British Medical Journal*. 2000;320:726–727.

13

Side hustles and interests beyond medicine

INTRODUCTION

In recent years, there has been a noticeable rise in doctors and surgeons pursuing interests beyond traditional clinical practice. Whether driven by personal passion, the desire for professional diversification, or the need to supplement income in an era of increasing financial pressures, more clinicians are embracing "side hustles" as part of their professional and personal development.

Beyond financial motivations, these alternative pursuits can serve as valuable outlets for creativity and self-expression. Engaging in activities outside of medicine has been shown to enhance overall well-being, foster resilience, and even improve workplace performance by promoting balance and perspective.

POPULAR SIDE HUSTLES AMONG CLINICIANS

1. **Social media and influencer activities**
   More and more doctors are using platforms like Instagram, YouTube, and podcasts to talk about health, well-being, and life in medicine. These channels allow clinicians to educate wider audiences, combat misinformation, and build personal brands. That said, being active online comes with responsibilities. The General Medical Council (GMC) provides clear guidance for those engaging in social media activities. The GMC advises,

   > *If you use social media to advertise your services, or use your professional position to promote or endorse any other services*

DOI: 10.1201/9781003537663-13

or products, you must be open and honest about any interests you have that may influence (or could be seen to influence) the recommendations you make.

Clinicians must also adhere to regulations from the Committee of Advertising Practice, Advertising Standards Authority, and Competition and Markets Authority to maintain transparency and professionalism online.

2. **Developing educational resources**
   Producing medical education content such as online courses, revision guides, or interactive workshops has become an increasingly popular venture. Advances in digital learning platforms have made it easier to reach a global audience, allowing clinicians to share expertise beyond traditional classrooms. These projects not only provide passive income but also contribute to the wider medical community by supporting learning and knowledge dissemination.
3. **Cosmetic procedures**
   Some doctors choose to broaden their scope of practice by offering aesthetic treatments like Botox or dermal fillers. While this can be a great way to diversify clinically, the GMC is clear that doctors should only work within their level of competence. That means having the right training, keeping skills up to date, and putting patient safety first at all times. For resident doctors especially, it's important to tread carefully. This usually means speaking with an educational supervisor, making sure the work doesn't clash with training requirements, and only practising in approved, properly regulated settings.
4. **Wellness services**
   Wellness-focused services, such as vitamin or mineral infusions, have become increasingly popular. For some clinicians, this work fits naturally with an interest in prevention and holistic care. However, it's not without its responsibilities. Doctors still need to base what they offer on sound evidence, have appropriate indemnity in place, and make sure they're complying with relevant regulations. Just because something is marketed as "wellness" doesn't mean the usual professional standards no longer apply.
5. **Creative and entrepreneurial pursuits**
   Not all side projects have to be clinical. Many doctors branch out into creative or entrepreneurial areas like writing fiction, running blogs, launching online projects, or investing in property. These pursuits can provide extra income, but just as importantly, they can offer a mental break from the pressures of clinical work. As long as these activities do not undermine professional responsibilities or public trust, they can be a healthy and fulfilling way for doctors to explore interests beyond medicine.

BALANCING MEDICINE AND SIDE PURSUITS

Finding time for additional pursuits within a demanding surgical or medical career can be challenging. Success often lies in strategic time management, setting realistic goals, and maintaining flexibility. Starting small, perhaps dedicating 30–60 minutes a week to a new project, can make the process manageable. Over time, these small, consistent efforts can evolve into meaningful and fulfilling ventures.

It is equally important to approach these interests with self-compassion. During particularly busy or stressful periods, it may be necessary to pause or scale back. Viewing side hustles as opportunities for personal growth rather than obligations helps maintain balance and prevents burnout.

LESSONS AND PROFESSIONAL CONSIDERATIONS

Engaging with side projects can cultivate valuable transferable skills such as leadership, communication, and innovation which in turn enrich one's medical career. They also promote longevity in the profession by reinforcing a sense of autonomy and purpose.

However, doctors must remain mindful of their professional responsibilities and the GMC's overarching guidance:

> *Whatever work you're doing outside of your day job, you need to act with honesty and professionalism, maintain confidentiality, ensure you have appropriate indemnity, and work within your sphere of competence.*

When approached thoughtfully, side hustles can complement rather than compete with one's medical career, supporting personal fulfilment, financial stability, and continued professional excellence.

BIBLIOGRAPHY

General Medical Council. *Using social media as a medical professional.* London: General Medical Council; 2024. Available from: https://www.gmc-uk.org/professional-standards/professional-standards-for-doctors/using-social-media-as-a-medical-professional/using-social-media-as-a-medical-professionalGoogleScholar

Rimmer A. Can I have a side hustle as a doctor?. *British Medical Journal.* 2024;385:q1136. https://doi.org/10.1136/bmj.q1136 (Published 03 June 2024).

14

General surgery in the age of social media

INTRODUCTION

Over the past two decades, social media has become an integral component of daily life. In most Western countries, more than 90% of adults have access to a smartphone, enabling continuous and immediate engagement with digital platforms. This widespread connectivity has transformed the way individuals communicate, access information, and form opinions, including within healthcare.

Surgeons, like the wider population, have increasingly adopted social media for both personal and professional purposes. Studies report that a significant proportion of surgeons use at least one social media platform, with user rates varying depending on specialty, seniority, and platform type. LinkedIn, Facebook, Twitter/X, Instagram and WhatsApp remain the most used platforms, particularly among younger surgeons and trainees who use these tools for education, networking, advocacy, and professional visibility.

While social media platforms offer significant opportunities ranging from patient education to global collaboration, their ubiquitous use also introduces complex challenges. Issues of professionalism, patient confidentiality, misinformation, and boundary management are increasingly relevant in an era where professional identity is often publicly visible and permanently recorded.

DOI: 10.1201/9781003537663-14

SOCIAL MEDIA IN SURGICAL PRACTICE: OPPORTUNITIES AND RESPONSIBILITIES

Commonly used social media platforms among surgeons include Twitter/X, Instagram, Facebook, WhatsApp, and LinkedIn. Each platform serves different functions: Twitter/X facilitates rapid academic discussion and advocacy; Instagram offers visual storytelling and patient-facing education; LinkedIn supports professional networking; WhatsApp enables private group communication and informal learning. However, these platforms are also easily accessible to patients and the public. Surgeons must therefore be mindful of their influence and visibility. Building an online presence that prioritises education and transparency over overt self-promotion is essential. While social media can support practice marketing, it also risks fostering unrealistic expectations regarding outcomes, particularly when surgical results are selectively presented or heavily curated. Surgeons may increasingly find themselves re-educating patients whose expectations have been shaped by filtered images, testimonials, or non-evidence-based claims.

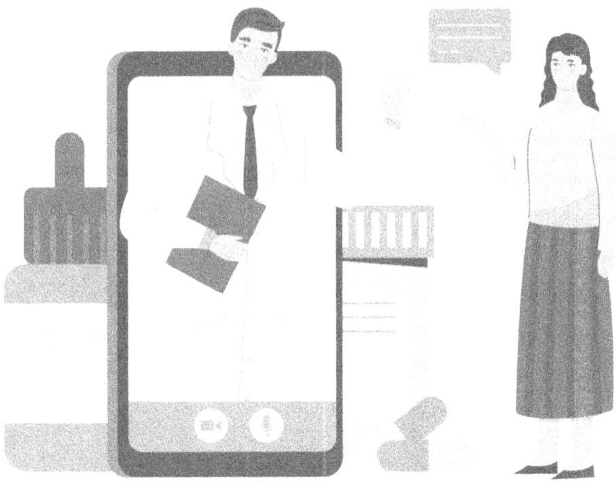

PROFESSIONAL EDUCATION AND TRAINING

Social media has emerged as a valuable adjunct to traditional surgical education. Platforms such as YouTube, Twitter/X, and WhatsApp are widely used for sharing operative videos, discussing complex cases, and disseminating new research. This informal learning environment allows surgeons and trainees to engage in continuous professional development beyond geographical and institutional boundaries. Virtual journal clubs, online case discussions, and live-streamed conferences facilitate rapid dissemination of best practices and foster an international learning community that complements formal training pathways.

MENTORSHIP AND PROFESSIONAL SUPPORT

Social media has redefined mentorship in surgery by enabling connections that were previously limited by geography, hierarchy, or institutional culture. This has been particularly impactful for women and underrepresented groups in surgical specialties who may lack access to same-sex or culturally aligned mentors within their own institutions. The #ILookLikeASurgeon movement exemplifies the power of social media to challenge stereotypes and promote diversity and role models. Originating as a grassroots campaign led by female surgeons, it highlighted the diversity of the surgical workforce and inspired global dialogue around equity, representation, and inclusion. Such initiatives demonstrate how social media can foster solidarity, encouragement, and professional identity formation.

GLOBAL COLLABORATION AND NETWORKING

Social media enables surgeons to connect with peers worldwide, facilitating collaboration on research projects, guideline development, and advocacy initiatives. Online professional communities allow for real-time exchange of ideas and experiences, contributing to the rapid evolution of surgical knowledge and practice.

PATIENT EDUCATION AND ENGAGEMENT

Used responsibly, social media can serve as a powerful tool for patient education. Surgeons can create patient-centred videos or infographics to share evidence-based information, clarify misconceptions and promote disease awareness. This can empower patients to engage more meaningfully in shared decision-making and may help reduce stigma associated with certain conditions or procedures.

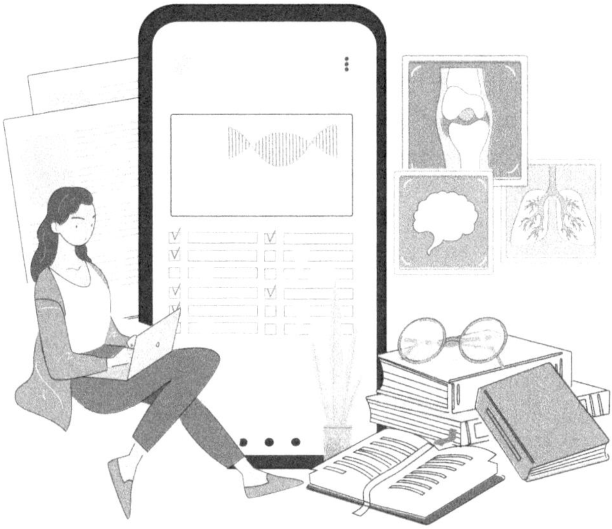

PRACTICE MARKETING AND VISIBILITY

Social media also provides a cost-effective platform for practice promotion and visibility. When conducted ethically and transparently, it can enhance public awareness, generate referrals, and highlight areas of expertise. However, marketing activities must remain consistent with professional standards and avoid sensationalism or misleading claims.

RISKS AND PITFALLS OF SOCIAL MEDIA USE

Despite its benefits, social media poses significant risks for surgeons. Awareness and proactive management of these risks are essential for both enthusiastic users and cautious observers.

MISINFORMATION AND UNREALISTIC EXPECTATIONS

The open and unregulated nature of social media allows misinformation to spread rapidly. Health-related falsehoods such as anti-vaccination narratives or exaggerated claims about surgical outcomes can negatively influence patient decision-making and clinical care. Heavily edited images and curated success stories contribute to unrealistic beauty standards, fuelling dissatisfaction and increasing demand for cosmetic procedures, particularly among younger populations. Research has demonstrated an association between social media use, reduced self-esteem, body dysmorphia, and an increased inclination toward aesthetic interventions.

PATIENT PRIVACY AND CONFIDENTIALITY

Sharing patient-related content, even when anonymised, carries the risk of breaching confidentiality. Violations of privacy regulations such as General Data Protection Regulation (GDPR) can result in serious legal, professional, and reputational consequences. Surgeons must exercise extreme caution when posting clinical material and ensure that informed consent is explicit, documented, and comprehensive.

UNPROFESSIONAL CONDUCT AND "MEDUTAINMENT"

Content that trivialises patient experiences, sensationalises procedures, or prioritises entertainment over education – often referred to as "medutainment" – can undermine public trust in the profession. Inappropriate posts may also attract regulatory scrutiny and damage both individual and institutional reputations.

BLURRED PROFESSIONAL BOUNDARIES

Direct interaction with patients on personal social media accounts or providing individualised medical advice online can blur professional boundaries. This may create false expectations, expose surgeons to medico-legal risk, and compromise the integrity of the patient–physician relationship.

SELECTION OF UNQUALIFIED PRACTITIONERS

Patients may choose surgeons based on online popularity rather than credentials, training, or outcomes. This phenomenon has contributed to the rise of surgical tourism and, in some cases, engagement with unqualified or uncertified practitioners, increasing the risk of poor outcomes.

REGULATORY GUIDANCE: THE GMC PERSPECTIVE

The General Medical Council (GMC) emphasises that professional standards apply equally online and offline. Identifying oneself as a doctor on publicly accessible platforms carries responsibility, as content may be perceived as representative of the profession as a whole.

Key principles outlined by the GMC include the following:

- Acting honestly and transparently, including declaring conflicts of interest
- Maintaining patient confidentiality and professional boundaries
- Providing appropriate context and evidence when discussing health-related issues
- Recognising that anonymous or private communications may become public
- Understanding that fitness-to-practise concerns arising from social media activity may be investigated

Medical professionals retain rights to freedom of expression and privacy; however, these rights must be balanced against the potential impact on patients, colleagues, and public trust.

USING SOCIAL MEDIA RESPONSIBLY IN SURGICAL PRACTICE

While social media provides a myriad of benefits, it also presents risks related to patient confidentiality, professionalism, and ethical conduct. This section outlines how surgeons can effectively use social media while upholding the standards of medical practice, ensuring a positive impact on their profession and patient care.

MAINTAINING PROFESSIONAL BOUNDARIES

While social media enables rapid communication, accepting patient "friend" requests or engaging through personal accounts is strongly discouraged. Such interactions risk exposing personal information and undermining the traditional professional relationship between surgeon and patient.

RESPECT FOR COLLEAGUES AND PROFESSIONAL CONDUCT

Social media provides unprecedented opportunities for peer support, particularly for surgeons working in remote or rural settings. Respectful discourse, collegiality, and support for diversity should underpin all professional interactions online.

SURGEON AS PATIENT ADVOCATE AND RESOURCE

Given the vast amount of health information available online, surgeons have an important role as patient advocates. By sharing accurate, evidence-based content and countering misinformation, surgeons can help patients navigate complex and often contradictory online narratives.

Although patients spend relatively little time with healthcare providers each year, they spend thousands of hours engaging with others online. Social media therefore represents a valuable supplementary channel for communication and education when used appropriately.

PROFESSIONALISM AND PUBLIC TRUST

Professionalism remains the foundation of the social contract between surgeons and society. As highlighted by GMC guidance, content authored by individuals identifying as doctors is likely to be taken on trust. Surgeons must therefore ensure that their online presence reflects integrity, accountability, and respect for the profession.

CONCLUSION

Social media is no longer optional in modern surgical practice; it is an enduring and influential component of professional life. When used thoughtfully, it offers powerful opportunities for education, mentorship, advocacy, collaboration, and patient engagement. However, these benefits are accompanied by significant ethical, legal, and professional responsibilities. Surgeons must embrace the potential of social media while maintaining professionalism, safeguarding patient trust, and upholding regulatory standards. By acting as responsible content experts and role models, surgeons can help shape a digital environment that supports high-quality care, informed patients, and a resilient surgical profession.

BIBLIOGRAPHY

BMA Ethics Department. *Social Media, Ethics and Professionalism*. London: British Medical Association.

Chretien KC, Azar J, Kind T. Physicians on Twitter. *Journal of the American Medical Association*. 2011;305(6):566–568.

European Union. General Data Protection Regulation (EU) 2016/679 of the European Parliament and of the Council of 27 April 2016 on the protection of natural persons with regard to the processing of personal data and on the free movement of such data (General Data Protection Regulation). *Official Journal of the European Union*, 2016; L119: 1–88.

General Medical Council (GMC). *Good Medical Practice*. London: GMC; 2013 (updated 2024).

General Medical Council (GMC). *Using Social Media as a Medical Professional*. London: General Medical Council; updated regularly. Available from: GMC guidance documents.

Kung JW, Wigmore SJ. How surgeons should behave on social media. *Surgery (Oxford)*. 2020;38(10):623–626.

Luc JGY, Stamp NL, Antonoff MB. Social media in the mentorship and networking of physicians: Important role for women in surgical specialties. *American Journal of Surgery*. 2018;215(4):752–760.

Pew Research Center. *Social Media Use in Healthcare Professionals*. Washington DC: Pew Research Center.

Royal College of Surgeons of England. *Professional Standards and Regulation in Surgery*. London: RCS England.

Scott KR, Hsu CH, Johnson NJ, et al. Integration of social media in emergency medicine residency curriculum. *Annals of Emergency Medicine*. 2014;64(4):396–404.

UK Government. *Data Protection Act 2018*. London: The Stationery Office.

Ventola CL. Social media and health care professionals: Benefits, risks, and best practices. *Pharmacy and Therapeutics*. 2014;39(7):491–520.

15

The future of general surgery: Innovation, technology, and transformation

INTRODUCTION

General surgery is at the forefront of a technological transformation. Advances such as artificial intelligence (AI), robotic-assisted surgery (RAS) and novel pharmacological therapies are reshaping surgical practice and the way surgical care is delivered. At the same time, surgeons are caring for increasingly complex and co-morbid patient populations, all while global disease patterns and medical advances continue to evolve.

Training in general surgery has also changed, with greater subspecialisation and an expanding role for multidisciplinary and technology-assisted care. While these developments present exciting opportunities, it is essential that patient-centred care remains paramount. Future surgical practice must prioritise safety, equity, and accessibility to meet the needs of changing populations. This chapter outlines key emerging technologies in general surgery and explores their implications for future practice.

DOI: 10.1201/9781003537663-15

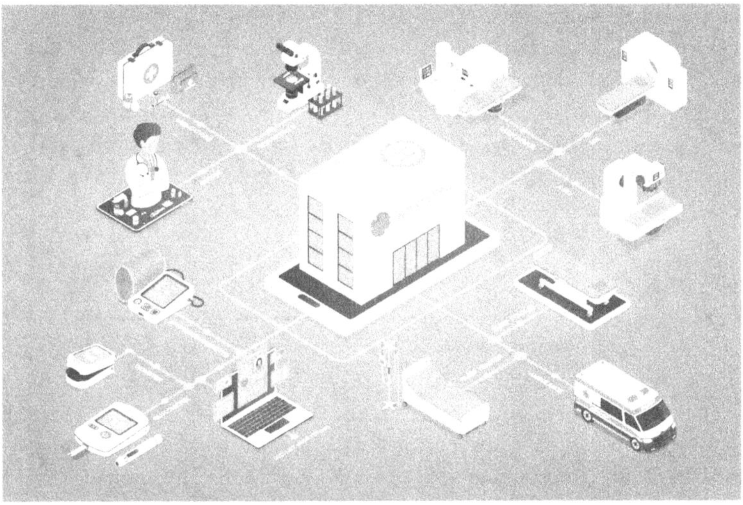

INNOVATION AND DEVELOPMENT OF NEW TECHNOLOGIES

Surgical innovation refers to the development and implementation of new techniques surgery which are designed with a focus on improving patient outcomes and enhancing surgical practice. The IDEAL framework was introduced to describe stages of innovation in surgery and standardise reporting of new innovations (Idea, Development, Exploration, Assessment, and Long-Term Study). Innovations may first begin with proof-of-concept studies or case studies, which may be scaled up to prospective studies or clinical trials to assess these techniques on a wider population.

Innovation may be individually driven or collectively driven. Innovations may arise from a single surgeon introducing a new technique or technology that they believe to be superior to the current status quo, or traditionally through surgical research and technological innovation supported by government or private infrastructures. Each variant may have their benefits and downfalls. While individual innovations may be faster and have a direct impact on clinical practice, under regulation and difficulties with "scaling up" may be encountered. Surgical research and clinical trials form the mainstay and gold standard of evaluating new innovations, although some of the drawbacks include resistance to changes in large healthcare systems. There may be limits to the speed of innovation based on funding limitations of healthcare systems and research. However, the NHS and institutions worldwide have a duty to support and encourage advancements. This is often done through education and training via programmes such as the NHS England Clinical Entrepreneur Training Programme, or through incubator organisations or competitions which seek to encourage wider adoption of successful innovations. Regardless, surgical innovators and institutions must recognise the importance of clinical governance and risk to patients when implementing new technologies or techniques in their clinical practice.

ADVANCES IN MEDICINE AND PHARMACOLOGY

Developments in medicine, radiology, and pharmacology are having a significant impact surgical practice. The use of pharmacological methods such as weight-loss medications has changed the landscape and practice of bariatric surgery, with the increasing uptake of glucagon-like peptide 1 (GLP-1) receptor agonist medications supporting non-operative weight loss. The practice of surgical oncology has also transformed with the introduction of neo-adjuvant therapies, targeted therapies, immunotherapy and hormonal treatment. Neoadjuvant therapy delivered typically through chemotherapy, radiation or a combination before surgical intervention can reduce the tumour burden to such an extent that, in some cases, surgical resection may no longer be deemed necessary. These are just contemporary examples of medical management shaping operative practice, and as new innovations in medicine and pharmacology are introduced, the landscape of surgery may change permanently.

The introduction of regenerative medicine and cell-based therapies have the potential to change the way surgeons practice. Preventative medicine such as vaccines can change disease landscapes, which can influence operative mixes. Improved understanding of the genetic basis of disease, alongside developments in genomic medicine, is also changing clinical practice. These advances allow earlier identification of individuals at risk of certain conditions and more accurate prediction of disease progression. As a result, surgeons will increasingly play a role in shared decision-making around preventative strategies, including risk-reducing surgery which will fundamentally transforming how surgical care is planned and delivered.

Beyond medical treatment, advances in minimally invasive techniques such as interventional radiology and endoscopy have changed the management of many conditions, enabling quicker recovery and improved patient outcomes.

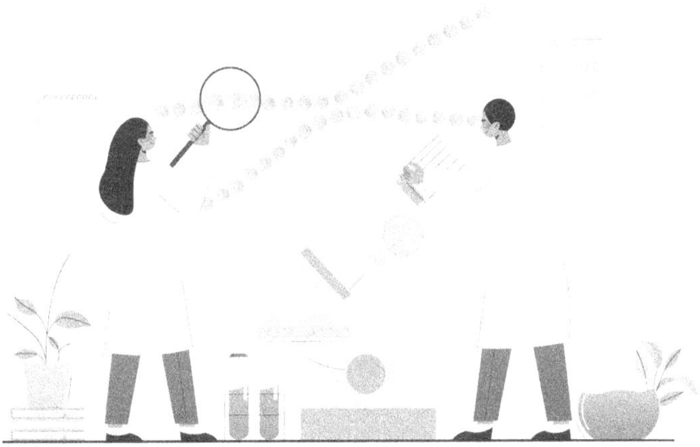

MINIMALLY INVASIVE SURGERY

Minimally invasive techniques such as laparoscopy and endoscopy are growing in popularity, and new indications are being introduced year-on-year. Although this is not a new development, new techniques and technologies are being introduced to make performing these procedures safer and more effective. Procedures which once required larger incisions and long recovery times have now become day procedures, and this has in turn led to shorter hospital stay and better operative outcomes. These have a knock-on effect on surgical care delivery, and the rise of day-surgery or ambulatory-surgery has changed the way hospitals work.

ROBOTIC-ASSISTED SURGERY

RAS is a relatively recent advancement that builds on established minimally invasive techniques, enabling surgeons to perform complex operations with greater precision, control, and dexterity. Compared with traditional open surgery and some laparoscopic approaches, RAS is associated with faster recovery, reduced post-operative pain, fewer wound complications, and minimal blood loss.

Surgical platforms such as the da Vinci Surgical System provide high-definition three-dimensional visualisation with magnification, enhanced instrument articulation, tremor filtration, and improved ergonomics, all of which can increase surgical accuracy and operator control. Newer robotic systems have since entered clinical practice, including Hugo™ RAS (Medtronic), which uses an open-console design, Dexter® (Distalmotion), which integrates robotic and conventional laparoscopic surgery at the operating table, and platforms developed by Cambridge Medical Robotics (now CMR Surgical), such as the Versius® system, designed to improve flexibility, portability, and access to robotic surgery. Beyond general surgery, robotic technology is now integral to several specialties, including urology (particularly prostatectomy), gynaecology, cardiothoracic surgery, colorectal surgery, and head and neck surgery, with ongoing expansion into additional surgical fields.

Looking ahead, continued advances in imaging integration, AI, and machine learning may allow increasing levels of automation and decision support. While fully autonomous robotic surgeons remain a distant prospect, robotic technology is already transforming surgical practice and is likely to play an increasingly central role across multiple surgical specialties.

ARTIFICIAL INTELLIGENCE

AI is a subset of computer driven machine learning which allows rapid and iterative processing of large datasets to support surgical processes. There is significant potential for the use of AI throughout surgical specialities.

In pre-operative planning, AI powered tools can support personalised medicine and patient-centred care and discussions. AI tools can also be used for prognostication and patient decision-making with operative suggestions tailored to patient choice.

In the operating room, AI algorithms applied to surgical robots or technologies can anticipate outcomes and support surgeons in identifying cancers intra-operatively with computer vision. AI can also support post-operative care through efficient patient monitoring – identifying patients at high-risk of deterioration at an early stage to allow direct intervention. AI can also support surgical education and training, and patient education. Gains in speed and process workflows can allow a safer, data-driven surgical practice which can put the patient first.

Big data

Data has a vital impact on patient care. Data on patient care, outcomes and safety can be used to drive decision-making in an evidence-based fashion through research and analysis. Data can also be employed in ensuring healthcare providers meet key quality metrics and outcome measures that can influence general surgery practices in terms of procedures and forward planning. In order to drive innovation, big data can be analysed via AI techniques to develop prognostication or support personalised medicine. Nevertheless, there are substantial regulatory and information governance considerations when it comes to the use of patient data.

3-D PRINTING

Additive manufacturing, also known as 3-D printing, has great potential in surgical fields. 3-D printing technologies can provide highly personalised implants for patients or even support surgical planning for complex approaches. For example, 3-D printing can be used in transplant surgery, through the development of bioengineering or bio-printing to generate organs or tissue to support patients requiring transplants.

VIRTUAL REALITY AND AUGMENTED REALITY (AR)

Virtual reality (VR) and AR can provide high-fidelity simulation training to train future surgeons to perform simulated procedures. These technologies can improve patient outcomes through ensuring standardisation of training and increase equity of access. VR and AR can also support planning of surgical approaches, and as these technologies continue to develop, future surgeons may find these education approaches integrated into the surgical training curriculum.

Culture shifts in medicine and surgery

In addition to technological advances, the future of general surgery is shaped by broader cultural changes in medicine and surgery. Shifting patient demographics, particularly ageing populations, have led to increased demand for surgical services. This has been discussed in detail in previous chapters.

General surgery has become increasingly subspecialised, with subspecialist surgeons facing greater demand as patients present with more complex co-morbidities. Clinicians are now expected to develop expertise in specific procedures, which may lead to improved outcomes for selected conditions. This shift is reflected in evolving training pathways and the expansion of recognised subspecialties.

As surgical practice becomes more specialised, the organisation of care has also changed. Within the NHS, this is reflected in the adoption of a "hub-and-spoke" model, where complex sub-specialist care is delivered in regional centres, while local hospitals provide initial assessment and referral to central hubs.

REGULATORY AND LEGAL IMPLICATIONS

Notwithstanding the fast pace of technological advancements in general surgery, patient safety must remain at the core of care delivery. There are significant risks in applying new and untested technologies to patient care, and these may harm patients instead of doing good. There are legal and regulatory requirements that must be fulfilled before a technology is used in patient care to ensure that new innovations are implemented safely and accountably. There must be adequate training and preparation of infrastructure for adoption of surgical innovations.

Implications for future surgeons

The changing landscape of general surgery has impacted surgeons, trainees, and healthcare infrastructures alike.

For surgical trainees, it is vital to maintain key operative skills and preparedness for training in new minimally invasive or robotic techniques. Although case mixes may shift in light of introduction of new surgical techniques, it is often vital to maintain one's general competencies and knowledge, especially about non-operative options for patients. There may be an expectation to sub-specialise in a field of one's choice in future.

For future surgeons, growth in subspecialities may result in increased multidisciplinary working and volume of work due to referrals and centralisation of care. Population dynamics may mean future surgical candidates are more frail or complex, and surgeons must be prepared to deal with a range of management options that may include medical and pharmacological advancements.

SKILLS SURGEONS OF THE FUTURE WILL NEED

General surgeons must be prepared for a rapidly evolving clinical landscape shaped by new technologies. Lifelong learning is essential: mastering new techniques often involves steep learning curves, but continual upskilling ensures surgeons can practice at their fullest potential. This requires a proactive, hands-on approach, including seeking practical experience, simulation, or robotic training both within and beyond formal curricula. Staying current with emerging technologies and research is equally important, as surgeons play a critical role in guiding innovation and shaping the development of new surgical tools.

Surgical trainees must maintain excellence in core operative skills, including emergency surgery, laparoscopic procedures, and endoscopy, while also developing skills in robotic surgery and emerging surgical technologies. Versatility and adaptability are vital to provide safe and effective care. While new technologies offer exciting possibilities, surgeons must remain objective, ensuring that all applications are evidence-based and safe. Beyond technical skills, there is an increasing need for expertise in acute and perioperative care to optimise outcomes in frail or complex patients. Conscious, outcomes-focused decision-making is key to maintaining high standards of care.

Collaboration with other disciplines, such as biotechnologists and engineers, is becoming increasingly important in developing and delivering advanced surgical care. Even as autonomous technologies emerge, surgeons remain essential in providing specialist oversight and ensuring patient safety. Above all, the human aspects of surgical care – that is, empathy, personalised care, and patient-centred decision-making – will continue to be central to excellent surgical practice.

CONCLUSION

General surgery faces an exciting future ahead. The core tenets of general surgery and management of emergency conditions and treatment of abdominal conditions remains key, yet surgeons must embrace the future through integrating new technologies, multidisciplinary collaboration and increasing training in new developments in order to remain future proof.

BIBLIOGRAPHY

Surgical Innovation, New Techniques and Technologies: A Guide to Good Practice. London: Royal College of Surgeons England; 2019. https://www.rcseng.ac.uk/-/media/Files/RCS/Standards-and-research/Standards-and-policy/Good-Practice-Guides/Old-documents/Surgical-Innovation-New-Techniques-and-Technologies.pdf

16

The calling of general surgery: A final word from the authors

General surgery is a discipline defined by its breadth, its rigour, and its profound impact on human lives. It is a journey that begins as early as medical school, weaving through a demanding series of stages designed not only to refine skill but also to identify those with unwavering dedication. The training is long, the learning deep, broad enough to shape clinicians of exceptional calibre, capable of meeting the intricate needs of modern patients.

The foundation years offer vital exposure to generalism, an essential phase in which the complexity of today's patients, whose needs often span multiple systems, calls for both versatility and precision. Rotational training in surgery, though intense, is deliberately structured to immerse trainees in diverse environments under varied mentorship, each stage contributing a new layer to the fabric of a future surgeon's expertise.

The path to becoming a general surgeon is marked by challenges and triumphs. It demands resilience, patience, and a constant willingness to grow. Yet, there is no equal to the moment when training gives way to independence, when the surgeon stands not as a trainee, but as a specialist, ready to serve with confidence and care.

Technical mastery alone does not define the general surgeon. At their best, general surgeons are agile thinkers and discerning decision-makers, their minds as incisive as their instruments, capable of navigating uncertainty with clarity and resolve. They are leaders who uplift their teams, nurture a culture of excellence, and drive forward the mission of their organisations. They are communicators who build trust with patients and

DOI: 10.1201/9781003537663-16

colleagues alike, ensuring empathy and integrity remain at the heart of their work.

Great general surgeons adapt with the times. They embrace evolving technologies, refine their techniques, and remain students of their craft long after formal training ends. Above all, they give back, passing on hard-earned knowledge with humility and purpose, ensuring the next generation is even better prepared for the road ahead.

Becoming a general surgeon is not merely a career choice, it is a calling. It demands hard work, sustained commitment, and a passion for service. Preparation is the cornerstone of success, and this textbook has been crafted to serve as your companion and guide, from the first sparks of interest in medical school to the honour of consultant practice. May it support and inspire you at every stage of the journey.

For Product Safety Concerns and Information please contact our EU representative GPSR@taylorandfrancis.com
Taylor & Francis Verlag GmbH, Kaufingerstraße 24, 80331 München, Germany

www.ingramcontent.com/pod-product-compliance
Lightning Source LLC
Chambersburg PA
CBHW070658290726
48947CB00041B/710
9781032882932